Of Health, Wealth, and Wisdom

A Practical Guide to Achieving Happiness

by Bernard Sherman Wiesel

Enlightened Path Publishing
Post Office Box 393
Lake Forest, CA 92609

A portion of book sales goes to Children International. (website: Children.org) This fine organization helps kids in need to get an education, which is essential to empower them and end the cycle of poverty.

Cover photo: Getty Images
Editor: Denise Bennett
ISBN: 978-1-7340802-1-6
Contact: Enlightened Path Publishing

Printed in U.S.A.

Acknowledgments

D ENISE, MY DAUGHTER, has been a constant help in guiding me through the process of writing and publishing my first book and now my second. Her knowledge, encouragement, and suggestions were invaluable and I am deeply grateful to her for that as well as for an endearing friendship.

I appreciate my wife, Rosalie, for her kindness in reading sections and giving her opinion. She was always willing to interrupt her day to help. She has provided insights I could not have imagined early on and demonstrates a rare love and loyalty for family.

Thanks to my parents, Alex and Mary, who worked diligently to provide guidance and inspire in an era when life was challenging.

My mother's identical twin, my Aunt Hilda (Bodan), was the light of my life. She and her husband, Uncle Josh, demonstrated strong traits of responsibility, integrity, and character; they became role models for me. The Bodans had two sons – the older was Burt. He became as a dear brother to me. We remained close our entire lives until he passed. Burt's widow, Doris Bodan, has my deep respect and love.

Mike McLean, a dear friend, has shared his guidance and wisdom with me over the years and I am very thankful for that.

I'm grateful too for my friend, Mitch Atlas – a quality individual. I send regards and thanks for a great friendship over many years.

Valuable lessons came to me through both of my children, David and Denise, who I thank for being in my life.

Lastly, I offer wholehearted appreciation for doctors, scientists, researchers, and other healthcare professionals who have given of themselves in such a way as to enhance our lives.

Contents

Introduction

"To him whose elastic and vigorous thought keeps pace with the sun, the day is a perpetual morning."

---- Henry David Thoreau

WELCOME TO MY book. Here is a destination that's set against a backdrop of knowledge, some words of wisdom, and a great deal of optimism. I invite you to have a little fun here. Get off the beaten path and discover something a little different. Look for possibilities that may offer some changes for the better. Is that too much to ask? (of course not.)

My focus in this book is to discuss various subjects in life that may have some connection for the reader, that reaches out to you and you may say, "Yes, I know about that," or "I have wondered about that," or "That happened to me."

I have often done the research, met with people who are knowledgeable on the subject, or read about the work or research of others, and gave credit where due.

Here are some of the standouts in this book: Correct Thinking; You *Can* Take It With You; Reincarnation: I Enjoyed the Ride, Let's Do It Again; Healing, Feeling, and the Mind; and The Seven Laws of Nature.

The basic theme here is to present a series of passages – brief chapters – which bring to readers ideas and information, with the specific objective of improving life. The thinking of writers and speakers, scientists, professors, philosophers, and religionists are shared to meet these objectives.

Do these ideas capture your interest? Know that I have deep respect for my readers... that I promise to make every effort to not waste your time, and to create a book that has some value for you.

Doing the research for this book enabled me to learn about relationships and how the Golden Rule is a constant application in improving life. I hope that in some way, readers can benefit from this book. A basic belief here is that lightness, laughter, and love bring about good health.

Some aspects of life as we seek happiness include the importance of meaningful relationships, and how gratitude is vital to good living and prosperity. Beliefs guide our actions, and those beliefs come from our perception. These things become our reality. You can have the blessing of good health and the joy of great wealth. Know that the quality of one's thinking is the key to life.

It can take many years to develop a good sense of humor in life, and not everyone is able to do it. People are so serious, thinking about their responsibilities; children to raise, duties at the job, bills to pay, and so on.

Some of the subjects written about in the book are the *Science of Happiness, Emotions, Beliefs, Power of the Mind, Perception, Relationships, Reincarnation,* and *Gratitude.* I have learned that one's attitude can have tremendous influence on the happiness that comes into their lives, and the people that grace those lives.

Life changes---that's a given---because there are many things that are outside of our control. But we need to deal with what has to be done. Unless your name is *Mary Poppins*, it is not going to materialize on its own. You will be the one to do it. *Step 1:* Identify the problem. *Step 2:* Determine what is needed to solve it. *Step 3:* Do it.

This is not luck. It is called WORK.

Right in your own hands is your destiny. The selection of your thoughts has the power to bring a harmonious and happy life right to your door. So let us begin!

Chapter 1

The Principles of Peace

W<small>E START WITH</small> a brief discussion about bringing peace and calm into your life. One may achieve a balanced mental position and a relatively stress-free life when they make much effort in this. "You can embrace a peaceful way of living," states Kathy Juline, author and life coach. Think about this: *What do I want in this life?*

Be very specific. As an example… if people disappoint you, decide what reaction you will take to remain in <u>calm detachment.</u> This detachment is a road to better mental and physical health. Think about this carefully. There is nothing so vital in this life as good health. Do you agree?

You should have a conscious sense of joy *and love* for your life. Mostly, we tend to ignore things. We think having joy or happiness or love will come automatically. Our attention goes to the details; the job, the children, household duties, etc. Of course.

But, there are individuals who are very effective in changing their lives by using self-talk; they write and use **specific statements that reflect things that they want in their life.** They use *affirmations.*

These persons are change agents for their own lives. They desire change and they will have it!

Here is an example of self-talk: "I want a calmness in my daily life. I need less emotional upheavals. I now establish gentle interaction with my children (or wife, husband, etc.). I desire loving thoughts; more peace and sweetness in this home. I clearly affirm these changes."

Your feelings here are very important. Affirmations need to come from your heart. Allow your feelings to surface; do not suppress them. Later, we will talk about affirmations and how important they are.

Life's Illusive Ingredient: Happiness

You can ask any person, "Are you happy in your life?" and there usually appears a quizzical look, followed by silence. People aren't really sure if they are happy. Of course, there are times when we are ecstatic about some event: gazing upon a new-born; looking into the face of a loved one; getting married; getting the career position we dream of.

The challenges in this life happen continually because that's how we grow. It is how we learn. I believe happiness is related to the amount of maturity that has developed in us. It's a series of events, like a round robin. We are born – as babies, we smile right away. And as we grow, we experience challenges and hardships. Lessons are being learned; we gain a bit of maturity.

Then there is some education that comes into the picture. Grade school and high school, and then there are decisions to make. One may be trained for a specific job or career; many people attend college or have other formal training. Working at a job will usually result in great experience and much maturity also.

Participating in some kind of labor in this world – the ability to provide a product or service to someone, and the beauty of being energetic and enthusiastic about life – is unquestionably a source of happiness.

True happiness appears fleeting until a person reaches 35 or 40 years, which may mean we find a loving companion and start a family, or we experience other social development and contentment.

Happiness Is A Personal Decision

Let me remind you of something you already know: **Your happiness is dependent upon *you!* You hold the power to determine your life.**

Unhappy people want to change events, conditions, their boss or coworkers, neighbors and family members – the list goes on and on. But they have it backwards. The first thing that needs to happen is to realize that <u>we</u> have to change, not others.

The world responds to your thought (about it) and the conditions in your life. Everything that happens to you happens *because of you.* Change the negative thoughts and moaning to **positive thinking**. Begin to appreciate <u>every situation and every person in your life</u>. This is a tall order... can you do it?

It might be the most difficult thing you have ever done, but your life will change. Neale Donald Walsch wrote, "All of life exists as a tool of your own creation." (from *Conversations with God)* He states further that the events of our lives are presented for us to decide about them. Walsch continues, "...we justify our lives through our experiences, and our experiences give us purpose."

If there is something going on in your life that you strongly dislike, think about changing it. If family or others will be affected by that change, you need to consider it carefully. Do your best to anticipate what will happen. How would *you* be affected by the changes you are proposing?

There is something else. When a person decides to be happy, they state it. They *affirm it.* Do not think that your statement is without importance or effect. The statements we utter are like declarations... like signals to the subconscious.

The truth is, you can direct your mind to modify any situation. Let me say that again. You can direct your mind to change any situation. You are in charge of you and what happens in your life. Of course, if you have family or others to consult with, then do that, with respect and cooperation. But you have a right to happiness... and the happiness you bring about is contagious!

Now, of course, action must be taken. List the steps you are going to take to improve your life. Here are some suggestions, but really, you should choose your own:

1) Make the decision to be happy and improve your life.

2) State that you deserve to be happy.

3) The fact that you are alive confirms your right to be happy.

4) When one asks how you are, try not to complain or whine.

5) Do not say what you *don't* want to happen. Say what you *do* want.

6) Stop saying life is awful. What comes out of your mouth is yours.

7) Find something good to say about every human in your life. If you can't find anything good, say nothing.

8) Lift your consciousness. Think positive (pleasant) thoughts; decide to live a rich, rewarding life; expect wonderful things to come into your life.

9) Read materials or books that help you find solutions to problems, aiming to improve daily life.

10) 10. Do different things; dress better, do more social activities, talk with neighbors, and modify your beliefs to embrace an expanded spirituality.

Decide with all emotionality and determination to be healthy and joyful each and every day, knowing that your words are powerful, because *you are powerful.* You are the star that the Creator made.

The Nature of Life. Study the nature of life and you will know the nature of happiness. Everything on earth vibrates. It is energy... and it is always in motion. Nothing remains the same.

One day you will find the beautiful and exciting discovery called *love.* Perhaps this has already happened for you. It's wonderful, isn't it? But it rarely lasts.

Happiness – joy – is the gift you have been given. But remember-----you have control as to what you do with expressing it. Happiness begins with your thoughts. Your thoughts will result in **1)** much happiness, or **2)** some happiness, or **3)** very little happiness. Here is an example:

"Boy, I have so much to do today; I'm worried. A lot can go wrong, I am sure of that. And that guy at work is a pain! He drives me nuts." (by Nervous Nellie)

"Well, I have a lot to accomplish. But I'm pleased that I have the energy to do it. I'm glad that my coworker will help. It'll probably be fun!" (by Smiling Sally)

You see that thoughts turn into words, and we have to be careful what we say.

<u>Experiment With Happiness.</u> Shall we have fun with an experiment? You have about 60,000 thoughts in a 24-hour period. Let's say you get a dollar for every positive thought or word you think... smiling, being kind or considerate, being polite, saying "thank you" or "I love you" to someone, etc.

Now add this. You *lose* a dollar for every negative thought or word... for every complaint, grievance, frown, mumble under your breath, etc. Let us say your positive to negative thought ratio is 3-1. Congratulations... you just earned yourself $30,000! You will have to pay a lot of tax to Uncle Sam, but you should net-out over $18,000. That's pretty good for a day's pay.

How To Be Happy

About fifty years ago, psychologists began to study the nature of happiness in human beings... and how to achieve more of it. Many people feel that a state of happiness does not truly exist, or if it comes around, it is a brief little spurt that does not last for long.

Then there is a group of humans that are good-natured; they smile a lot, get over their moods quickly, and are usually very sociable. Who are we talking about? *Babies!*

There is a wide variety in human beings as they respond to similar circumstances. In the exact same situation, some people are happy and others are sad or upset. Why this difference? People, according to psychoanalyst Erich Fromm, succeed at being happy in the same way they succeed at loving... *by building a liking for themselves.*

One needs to have a strong sense of self-worth, and a healthy amount of self-respect. One gains these traits by meeting personal goals and accomplishing things like graduating from school, meeting requirements in Scouting or other organizations, earning a college degree, learning to play a musical instrument, being in the theater or chorus, or securing a position in business.

Then there's the best thing in the world... having love in your life, and having people you care for deeply. Now that is an achievement. And if you have children and are a good parent, that is also an achievement and something to be proud of.

I have great respect for a man who specialized in happy and successful living. Raymond Charles Barker (1911-1988) addressed large audiences at New York's Lincoln Center, and is the author of several books on healthier, happier living. Some of these include *How to Be Healthy, Wealthy, Happy; Treat Yourself to Life; The Science of Successful Living; The Power of Decision.* I would urge you to do this: identify the problem. Like any project you want to succeed at, the first thing to do is to gain information, and state the desire you have. A library or book store provides information, but you must move on it. Take action!

Mental Nourishment. You remember that we have thousands of thoughts that enter our subconscious mind every day of our lives; twenty-four hours a day. We need them... we need to have ideas. Barker reminds us that ideas are as essential to our mind as food and water are to our physical body.

New ideas come into our consciousness to provide progress in our lives. We cannot stay the same. Whether we like it or not… whether we resist change or not, we are going to proceed on our path. Nothing stays the same for long.

We instinctively know when it's time to quit something and move on to something else. We have a built-in resistance to change but eventually, we have to give in. We frequently put things off until tomorrow or next week or next month. Who among us has not had the experience of procrastination?

We need to grow; ideas give us the ability to grow out of old habits and make room for the new.

Take a look at something that you have had in your life for a long time. Does it have value? Is it productive? Does it contribute to your happiness or self-worth? If not, consider replacing it with something new.

The human mind dislikes change. You may be in your comfort zone but ask, "How would I benefit from changing this?"

<u>Some definitions of Happiness.</u> Erich Fromm said that happiness is an achievement, brought about by a sense of being productive. Aristotle believed that happiness is obtained by being self-sufficient. When Timothy Dwight was president of Yale University, he said that happy people are those who think interesting thoughts. William McDougall, psychologist, said that one's level of happiness depends on the individual personality. Many older Americans say that happiness depends on staying busy, being able to work well, enjoying family and friends, and having various interests.

Unhappy people rarely blame themselves for their condition. The problem is their lousy job or their marriage, what fate dealt them, how their parents treated them, etc. They believe life is unfair. Usually they have nothing to give, in work, play, or relationships. Unhappy people clearly are those who criticize others, and they criticize them often. They have a great deal of blame to go around, attributing this to their misery.

Happiness and Health. These generally go hand-in-hand. Happy people do not become ill as often, and they recover more quickly. Those who indulge in anger, hate, fear, and guilt are subject to pain and suffering. But don't be afraid of your emotions. When things are fine, life is great; the mood is stable. And when challenges come around, these unpleasant emotions surface. As Thich Nhat Hahn says, "An emotion comes, stays for a while and goes away, just like a storm."

Emotions can be helpful if they point out problems that need to be addressed, and people work to solve those issues. Do not discount the importance of emotions.

I believe that the cause of all sickness is stress, the close cousin of negative emotion... while the sweetheart of good health is an active sense of humor; lots of laughs. Laughing is very important. It can keep you healthy.

Controlling Your Life. This is easier said than done. You decide that you want certain things or situations in your life. That seems normal, particularly at a young age. But as one matures, he thinks about his future and collects things--- cars, televisions, cell phones, etc. And when he has a family, he recognizes the requirements of modern society, such as a satisfactory credit rating or a strong work ethic – to be able to function in conventional ways and meet important responsibilities to attain one's goals.

Let's bring into discussion the subconscious mind. Everything that has ever happened to a person is because of the subconscious mind. The subconscious is the record of all that a person has experienced, from his first breath.

Let the person use the conscious to guide the subconscious to whatever is desired in one's life. The conscious mind is the controller; it is the decision-maker. Now make up your mind… what do you want? Reach high and dream big. Navigate the present and determine your future. *It is entirely up to you!*

The conscious mind will wake you up in the morning *if* you instruct it to do so. The command is given and then carried out by the subconscious. You go to the store to buy some items; you stop to fill up your vehicle with gasoline; you wave to a friend. These are acts of the conscious mind.

It is a hot day and you decide to go for a swim. It has been months since you last swam. You change into your bathing suit, walk to the diving board, take your steps, then execute a perfect, smooth dive. You remembered everything, thanks to the subconscious mind.

An Inside Job. When people are unhappy, they want to change the situation, conditions, or the people in their lives. But, they do not want to change themselves. They think *incorrectly* that it is someone else's fault. Not them. The only thing you can truly change is *you*. Happiness is an inside job.

The changes that have to occur involve modifying one's own behavior, such as adopting a better attitude about other people. There's an old expression that says, *everything that happens to you happens because of you.*

You can change any situation for the better, but first you need to ask yourself, "Do I really want to change?" A change requires effort. Mary Poppins is a wonderful story, but it is not reality.

Reality says if you want a raise, work hard and you may get one. Improving a situation takes a great deal of patience and commitment. I ask myself, "Do I really want to change this?"

If I want it different, I have to *make* it different. How do I do this? I need to find out the first sensible step in bringing about change. And---I need to take that step.

<u>You are responsible for your life.</u> This statement says that the individual has all the power they need to create the life they desire. I believe that we were created or evolved, then given freedom; freedom to choose. We are not robots. We are human beings with tremendous ability to make our choices.

We can choose habits for our daily life, foods that we eat, games we want to play, people we like to be with, and the way we earn our living. We choose the attitude we take into our workplace.

We live on this tiny planet in this immense universe and we seek knowledge and understanding. I ask these 5 questions: **1)** How did I get here? **2)** Why did I come here? **3)** Why is there so much pain in the world? **4)** Why don't people get along? **5)** What am I supposed to do here?

It starts with ideas. The human mind has thousands of thoughts and ideas every day. Most are unimportant; they pass through the mind with intense speed. These include comments you made, things you heard, conversations, events that occurred, and decisions you contemplate.

It is estimated that the average adult makes about 35,000 decisions each day. Cornell University researchers estimate we make over 200 decisions on food alone, every day.

To find answers, start with ideas. Each individual has ideas from the mind as well as information gained from listening to others, observing the media, reading, studying, and attending workshops and classes. This process – gaining wisdom – may take years and usually requires a person to be receptive; to keep an open mind.

One might say, "I accept the process of taking a look at another opinion or idea. I can decide if it has merit for me."

In finding ideas to improve one's life, it is essential to use these two basics: thinking and feeling. Weigh the ideas carefully. Consider your personal feelings and develop your system of beliefs. What we believe is extremely important, because it affects our behavior. It affects our thoughts, and that in turn affects our relationships. It affects our <u>life.</u>

Up and Down. There's an old joke called, *That's Good, That's Bad.* Two men meet who haven't seen each other in a while. It goes like this...

Henry greets his old pal and says, "Did you hear I got married?"
Bill says, "Oh, that's good."
Henry: "No, that's bad. She's a nag."
Bill: "Oh, that's bad."
Henry: "No, that's good. She's got a lot of money!"
Bill: "Oh, that's good!"
Henry: "No, that's bad. She won't give me a cent."
Bill: "Oh, that's bad."
Henry: "No, that's good. She bought me a big house!"
Bill: "Oh, that's good!"
Henry: "No, that's bad. The house burned down."
Bill: "Oh that's bad."
Henry: "No, that's good. She was in it!"

Good, bad, good, bad. This old skit has a timeless message. Just how does this life work? I will tell you. *The nature of life is variety.* Up, down, up, down. Nothing stays the same for long. Can you name anything that stays the same?

The nature of life is <u>change.</u> The only consistent factor in this life is **change.** Expect change. It will come to your door and enter. You may as well let him in.

We all have challenging emotional experiences from time to time. Anger, disappointment, sorrow, frustration. But---the sooner you get a smile on your face, the better. The sooner you decide to celebrate your life – to count your blessings, and express gratitude for the life you have – the better.

It is very possible that the people who give you the most trouble are your teachers. They are here to provide us with the lessons we need to learn. It is believed that the negative events frequently turn into blessings, perhaps for our highest good. The Chinese use the same word for *crisis and opportunity*.

In talking about change, here's an exercise you can try: I call it THE FRIENDLY UNIVERSE. This is about traffic. People are in a big hurry these days. They cut you off, change lanes suddenly without signaling, and tailgate. Instead of cursing or blowing your horn, be courteous. Wave people in when you can. And when they let you in, give them a *thank you* wave back. I give them a little smile, too. You are going to see drivers in shock. Make the commute a pleasant thing. Be kind to other drivers, and your angst level will reduce substantially. You will arrive safely and with a smile on your face! ~

Chapter 2

The Power of Thought

RESEARCH INDICATES THAT we have 50-60,000 thoughts every day. Things come into our lives as a result of our thinking.

Here's a little story: Jane works hard at her job. She accepts an invitation from Sheila, her friend, to do lunch together. Sheila says, "I'll pick you up in my brand new car." They enjoy the lunch and time together. Jane begins to think about a shiny new car with that *new car smell* and all those extra features. The more she thinks about it, the more she sees herself in her own new car.

Jane has a good credit rating and the purchase fits her budget requirements. She does some research and visits a car dealership. She takes a test ride; she makes the deal. The salesman hands her the keys. The act of purchasing the car is directly related to a large number of **thoughts** that have come to her mind, and imaging. Imaging is the process of making a visual representation.

We spend a great deal of time attempting to find answers in this life. We ask, "Why do bad things happen? Why must some children go hungry? Why are some lives so short while others live a long time?"

Why is not important. The nature of life on this planet is occasionally negative. There is no getting around that. I submit that we are here to deal with our experiences---good and bad---and learn from them. The *learning* is key.

It is very difficult to understand exactly what we are to learn in every situation. Many times, our greatest blessings are disguised as traumatic events.

The everyday experiences that sometimes occur were given point value according to their trauma potency, as created by Dr. Thomas Holmes, psychiatrist (1919-1989). The full list is 45 items. Here are just a few:

Event	Point Value
Change in sleeping habits	16
Change in schools	20
Spouse begins or quits a job	26
Trouble with in-laws	29
Foreclosure of mortgage or loan	30
Addition to the family	39
Retirement	45
Fired from work	47
Personal injury or illness	53
Divorce	73
Death of spouse	100

In every situation, there is potential for learning; behaviors are modified. Change always takes place. Humans grow. These events are a natural part of life. We learn to live with some new awareness and understanding. Very likely we will gain some sensitivity for others, and ourselves.

Vibrations

Every person has a vibration – a mental atmosphere – which is the result of all they have ever thought, said, and done... consciously or unconsciously. Every person has a perpetual attraction. It's how they look and carry themselves; how they act or think they should act; how they look in the mirror, dress, or brush their hair; how they deal with the emotions they experience.

Each person thinks thousands of thoughts consciously and unconsciously <u>every day.</u> We have countless reactions to all sorts of input. We may laugh or we may cry; we might get angry, frustrated, exasperated or become fearful. It doesn't let up. Welcome to life!

You may as well get used to it. Our emotions accompany every breath we take. Thoughts about events and our reactions to them are subjective. This explains our likes and dislikes to a large extent. This explains how we may like someone we have met, and dislike another. We meet one person, and for no apparent reason, we are captivated by them. Yet with another, again with no apparent reason, we have utterly no interest whatsoever.

But it relates to the individual's aura or vibration. Much has been written about how to be attractive to others. The best suggestion I've heard is, "Put a smile on your face."

I've discovered that I am unable to live this life without recognizing a strong aspect of what I term *spirituality.* I define spirituality as a conscious awareness of the presence of a Higher Being... of Universal Intelligence (Einstein's term), an Infinite Presence throughout... in every form, God.

Living a spiritual life may mean being aware of the Presence of God (or Spirit) as One to communicate with. Perhaps an individual connects with this Being in many ways throughout his life. He has deep feelings that relate to life's blessings and challenges. It is clear to me that this life is a mystery, but I accept that. There are a thousand things I cannot understand (make that *ten-thousand*). But I will not sit around and moan about my ignorance. I shall stand tall and give it my best shot... adding some determination to the deal, and then move forward.

Philosophers and writers, the great thinkers, have attempted to describe the Divine. This is a good thing. It means that we are not just robots or inert, vegetative objects. We are dynamic beings who dream, and analyze, and wonder.

It was the French philosopher, Voltaire, who said, "If there were no God, it would be necessary to invent him." We need the Divine. To think that human beings are here with no connection to something beyond this human plane... that we simply appeared here... is absolutely inconceivable to me. The concept of the physical without spiritual is without reality. Every form exists because of its essence; its *spirit.*

Thus, throughout these writings, I offer brief passages on the subject of how we might improve our lives, and how our days might be made better.

At times, I enjoy reading about someone's life. Every life is unique; special. I find them interesting and some are incredibly different.

Take Voltaire, for instance. His name was Francois-Marie Arouet. (1694-1778). A philosopher and French writer, famous for his wit, he was an advocate for freedom of speech and religion, and the separation of church and state. He was a large influence in the French and American revolutions. Here are a few of his famous quotes:

"I disapprove of what you say
but will defend to the death your right to say it."
"Judge a man by his questions rather than by his answers."
"God is a comedian playing to an audience
too afraid to laugh."
"We all look for happiness,
but without knowing where to find it:
like drunkards who look for their house,
knowing dimly that they have one."
"A witty saying proves nothing."
"God gave us the gift of life; it is up to us
to give ourselves the gift of living well."
"The most important decision you make
is to be in a good mood."
"Every man is guilty of all the good he didn't do."

Voltaire's father disapproved of his son's decision to become a writer. Voltaire criticized the government and spent time in prison, but vastly influenced the world in politics, religion, and philosophy. Here is another interesting fact: Voltaire gave America's founding fathers important concepts upon which to build a new form of government.

The Aim of Life

Sometimes we ask, "Just what is the aim of life?" To be happy. Is that some kind of goal? And how do we do that? Let us say there is a family that struggles. Do the children have all they need? These parents worry; they both work hard at their jobs. They work overtime; they are fragile and use coupons to save on food and other items. So, are they happy? Do they have time to enjoy their children?

A man by the name of Prentice Mulford lived in the 1850's. He was an author in California and wrote humorous essays. He looked for his fortune during the 1849 gold rush but eventually concentrated on spiritual matters. Mulford also contemplated the aim of life. He said we should try to get the most happiness out of life by living each day joyfully, to the fullest.

These may be the thoughts for all of us. We want blessed health, loving relationships, prosperity, control over our lives, a home, family, clothing and cars; the sweet pleasures that make life comfortable.

Our goal should be to exude happiness to such a degree that others welcome our presence; to be no one's enemy and everyone's friend. How on earth do we do that? Do your remember what Voltaire said? The most important decision you make each day is to **be in a good mood.**

I tried this recently for an entire day. I was really surprised. Some people liked my mood. Some people did not like my mood. They seemed to be in a bad mood simply because of my *good* mood. You know what that is about? I believe they were jealous. OR they had other problems or priorities that took precedence.

Now, we all want to achieve happiness. But it can be fleeting. And when someone else is happy and we are not, we may become jealous.

At times, we don't know what to do to achieve happiness. I am convinced that much of the problem relates to *personality.*

Personality is a combination of characteristics or qualities that form an individual's character. Here are two persons: **1)** A person has a sunny disposition that is very engaging. **2)** This individual is bad-tempered, contentious, and grouchy. Which would you rather be with?

How is personality formed? It takes the influence of experiences, some happy and joyous, other experiences were fearful, anxious, or disappointing... especially when we are very young. But as we grew older, we went to pre-school, or kindergarten. Then we learned competition. And we were taught to share things with others.

We developed; we learned to use sound principles of behavior; we discovered that when we were kind to others, they liked us.

Forgiving others is one of the keys to living a happy life. But before I can forgive someone else, I need to forgive myself. At the core of forgiving is grace – joy, and love are present. This process is not an easy one.

One of the most complicated and powerful spiritual tools is gratitude. How do we accomplish this? Start with a drink of water. In many parts of the world, people do not have fresh, clean drinking water. It's a simple concept, but we can be grateful if we have essential things like food and water.

A Discovery

I have recently discovered that I am not always perfect. It has not taken much to discover it. The truth is that I have suspected this for a long time. Since I was about seven years old.

Actually, my imperfections are on several levels. Intellectual, emotional, social, and maturity, for a start.

But a good habit I have worked on a lot is curiosity. I have wondered about things since I was about 8 or 9 years of age. My parents were patient, especially my father, who had a standard answer when I asked about something. He'd say, "Let's look it up in a book."

From that, I developed a strong interest in reading and learning about life's mysteries. Somewhere between age 8 and the present, beliefs formulated. Here are just a few:

1) We go through various stages so that we can learn about life. At times, the body appears to suffer disease as a result of life lessons or spiritual growth. Writers, philosophers, and scientists, such as Buddha, Plato, Plotinus, Spinoza, Kant, and Descartes said that inner thought affects/creates sickness or health.

2) There will be disappointments and we will learn that it is important how we react to them.

3) There is a vast difference between human beings, even people we are related to biologically.

4) Even though we cannot define it, the concept of *love* will become very important in our life. We will spend great time and effort expressing it.

5) The element of fear will, at times, encompass our thoughts and frighten us. However, this is designed to preserve and strengthen our lives.

6) The only thing we can be sure of in this life is *change*.

7) Over time, we seek a deep awareness of some kind of spirituality that develops a sensitivity about the Divine.

8) Most of us learn that what we truly concentrate on and deeply desire, we eventually achieve.

9) It seems that most people, who embrace some kind of religious belief, have good hearts and are caring individuals.

10) The strength, spirit, and power of one's life correlates to deeply-held beliefs that an individual develops over many years.

Beliefs are so very important. From beliefs we dream, think, act, and grow. The conscious mind is the decider – a device that sets thought in motion. The subconscious mind is the receiver; a place we store the events of our past. It's the library. All of the data since *day one* of your life is stored there. It is a recurring theme in these writings, and its importance cannot be overstated. We will revisit the subject in later chapters.

I Want to Drive a Car

Here's a little story – I've added them throughout the book just for fun. When I was around seven years old, I went with my father on a few of his business trips. He let me steer the car when I was nine. When I was twelve, I brought the car to him at work a few blocks away.

I was fourteen when Dad was working at the War Manpower Commission. A car was assigned to him; it had Federal license plates. I drove short trips with that car even though I did not have a driver's license!

When snow and ice came to Newark, I enjoyed skidding around in the Government Dodge with the stick-shift transmission.

In the building where we rented an apartment, our neighbor was a police officer named Mr. Doremus. We had a long talk about driving without a license; he said that he would not tell my parents, but I needed to stop driving illegally. I promised him I'd obey the law... *and I kept my promise.*

Chapter 3

Decisions, Decisions, Decisions,

YOU ARE IN New York City. You need a ride, so you hail a cab. But to get a cab in *the City* is not always easy.

A taxi pulls over and stops; you get in. The cabby says, "Where to, Ma'am?" Now it is your turn. You have to answer, but you're not sure. You think fast and say, "The Empire State Building." The driver says, "Yeah, 34th and 5th."

Decisions! The average adult makes about 35,000 decisions a day. You must have a sharp mind to be able to do that.

The act of deciding is basically a habit. As time goes on, it gets easier. Let's get back to our New York visit. You are on the 102nd floor of the Empire State Building; it is quite a view.

Later, you decide to go to Central Park, the Plaza, Lincoln Center; then grab a superbly delicious Kraut Dog at Nathan's. Next, you head for Times Square, then end your day at Katz's Delicatessen where Billy Crystal and Meg Ryan had lunch in the film, *When Harry Met Sally.*

Making a decision is using the mind to get some result. One knows what he wants and <u>assumes</u> he can get it. Do not let worry get in the way of what you want. Generally, life will respond to your decision IF YOU HAVE CONFIDENCE that it is truly what you want *and you are willing to work for it.*

If deep inside of you there is worry, fear, or doubt, it probably will not work. You may sabotage your efforts with statements like, "I'll probably fail." "I'm too old to accomplish that." "It's probably above my ability level." "I can't afford that."

No great event happens by chance, states Raymond Charles Barker (1911-1988). It is caused, he said, by decisive thinking. If you really want to give power to your ideas, write them down.

The Journal Habit

I have had the habit of writing in a journal for many years. I enter my thoughts as well as passages from articles or books and other resources. What does this do? It provides me with ideas that I might use sometime in the future. I can alter my lifestyle, habits, and procedures... something I would adopt to improve life in some way, to make an acceptable change.

Today, for instance, I am writing about *Good Health, True Wealth.* Good health is taken for granted by most young people. They have this gift. The young don't even think about it. It is theirs. Then come the challenges of growing older. It is true that many people have excellent health their entire lives. That certainly is a blessing.

It is smart to take care of our bodies if we are to live long and healthy lives. We need nourishing food, proper rest, exercise, and good (right) thinking. Thinking good thoughts is very important for the care of our body. Do not think for a moment that this is unimportant.

Every act, every event, every decision that you make is preceded by thinking and hopefully, by *right* thinking. By right thinking I mean, thoughts that are free of anger or upset... nervousness and worry. If one is negative, he is likely to make a poor or inappropriate decision. Make your choices when you are calm and peaceful. In the thinking process, feelings are extremely important. Feelings can affect our decisions, and our health.

Longevity. Humans are designed to live 100 years. In some cases, they can extend life by continuing to grow and with a positive outlook. Research shows that an enriched environment expands the cognitive and spatial development of the brain. Positive mental expression usually draws healthy and enduring lifestyles. An individual who has an agreeable personality would very likely have a stable environment and positive experiences.

But living this life usually means strains and stresses, and that equates to a gradual erosion of one's good health. Most humans experience some health challenges as they reach their 70's, 80's, 90's and beyond. Isn't it wonderful that science and technology enable us to enjoy better living and longer life? In the 1700's, the life expectancy was 25; in the 1800's, it was 47; in the 1900's, 75. Now, in the 2000's, human beings are expected to live 120 years!

Now, I am not denying the impact of *pain* in our lives. It does occur. But years of study and empirical research –

analyzed quantitatively or qualitatively – gives me confidence that our thought processes have great influence on our health.

The Placebo Effect. A placebo is an inert substance or treatment. These can be tablets (made from sugar and distilled water), fake surgery, or other procedures. It is a remarkable phenomenon that can improve a patient's condition simply because the person **has the expectation that it will heal them.**

In an experiment, there is a test group. Then there is the control group, which is used as a benchmark to measure the results of a drug or treatment on the other group. In some studies, a "fake" or imagined shot or pill or procedure results in a physical change in the body. This is called, *the placebo effect...* and it is a testament to the power of the mind. It has been used successfully in improving one's health.

A research study in 2002 at Baylor School of Medicine in Waco, Texas, involved knee surgery to treat pain. Patients were divided into three groups. In the first group, Dr. Moseley shaved the damaged cartilage. In the second group, he flushed out the knee joint. In the third group, the doctor performed no surgery whatsoever.

The first two procedures are standard treatment for arthritic knees. All three groups were prescribed the same postoperative care. The results were shocking. The two groups that received surgery improved as expected. **But the placebo group improved just as much as the other two groups!**

One of the participants in the *Placebo Group*, Tim Perez, walked with a cane before the surgery. Afterward, he was able to walk without the cane... and play basketball with his grandchildren. Tim was interviewed on the Discovery Health Channel. He said, "In this world, anything is possible when you put your mind to it. Your mind can work miracles."

Here is a mathematical formula. Good health = true wealth.

More On Decisive And Correct Thinking

Nothing is so important as sound decisions and correct, *balanced* thinking. Be clear about what you want in this life. All of our thoughts, actions, and expressions derive from and give off energy. *Make use of this energy!*

Scientifically speaking, there are many forms of energy. There is electrical energy, heat energy, chemical, radiant, and kinetic energy, to name a few. But what other type of energy is there? Here is an example of bringing energy to a situation that was somewhat tense.

In my neighborhood is an elderly man who appears lonely and hostile about life. Recently, our postman accidentally delivered his mail to me. I really didn't want to go over to his house – he is always so grumpy and complaining. But I knew I had to go. So, I rang the doorbell, and after a long while he opened the door *just enough*. He peered at me. Right then I decided to add some humor to the situation...

"Good afternoon. I am your new postman!" Realizing his mail was delivered to my house he said, "Doesn't the postman know my address?" He grumbled a little, then saw my big smile, and to my surprise, he returned it! After a little chat, we both said cheerful good-byes. Energy was brought to the meeting with a bit of lightness and fun. In all these years, he has rarely called me by my first name. But as I left he said, "Thank you, Berney."

I share this to show how our actions impact others. In that moment, my neighbor needed kindness and my gesture lifted his spirits. That was a day we'll both remember.

Just how does energy work? Where does it come from? I can tell you. *First, be in control. You decide what is going to happen.* In the scene above, I did not care to hear the man complain about the United States Postal Service. I decided to

APPLY A LITTLE HUMOR TO THE SITUATION and mollify the negatives.

People rarely reject humor, so I threw a little at him. I brought **positive energy** to this scene, and <u>I chose the kind of situation it was going to be.</u> Now if you want to argue or join in grumpiness, go for it. You are in charge. Whether it is a relationship, a business meeting, talking with your neighbor, or a clerk or food server, or any other encounter. You can choose the type of energy you will use and the experience you want to have.

Let's Talk About Consciousness

First, let's define *consciousness.* It is awareness of the world and all there is. It is a state of being awake and aware of one's surroundings. It is being perceptive; having thoughts and feelings. Here are some synonyms: mindfulness, attention, knowing, and observation. Consciousness enables us to create, learn, and connect with others, assisting with our social nature. It gives us power to make decisions… to learn, analyze, adapt, and to choose.

As human beings, we have tremendous power. No, we aren't ants. We can't carry many times our body weight. But humans can create their lifestyles, their health, their social and emotional experiences; they create their successes and their failures. Let me say that again:

Humans create their successes and their failures.

So much depends on experience and what we were told; how we were influenced, and the formation of our beliefs. Do you believe that you are a valuable person on this earth and that you have much to offer the world? That is the first step. To develop a strong sense of self. If you think that you aren't worth much – that you don't deserve a good partner or much income, or that you must struggle in your life – then that is probably what you are going to experience.

One needs a positive attitude to bring success into life. SAY THIS: *I am a worthy person. I deserve to have a good job. I have ambition; I will have a nice house/apartment, a nice car, money to buy things and go places. I am willing to work to get the things that make my life joyful and pleasant.*

Now that is called an affirmation. It is a statement affirming something that you want in your life, perhaps a deep feeling within you. I have used affirmations for a long time. This type of action is based on drawing from *within*, not so much from *without*.

The *within* draws thoughts, feelings, actions, hopes and dreams of one's consciousness, while the *without* is that which the brain recognizes as sensory stimuli through seeing, hearing, smelling, touching, and tasting.

Perhaps it is an awareness of power. Within yourself, you have a feeling, a desire, or a dream. It comes from within. The power then transforms into action… action such as signing up for a class, going on a trip or vacation, buying a house, getting a new apartment, taking steps to find a better job, registering to vote, going on a diet, or writing a book.

But remember that all of the events of our lives begin with **a thought.** You could have created it or this might be your intuition. Intuition is having understanding without conscious reasoning; something that just comes to you. One way or the other, I would advise a bit of self-talk. Try saying this: "Welcome, inspired thoughts… come to me." By doing this, you are inviting your intuition to guide and advise you. ~

Chapter 4

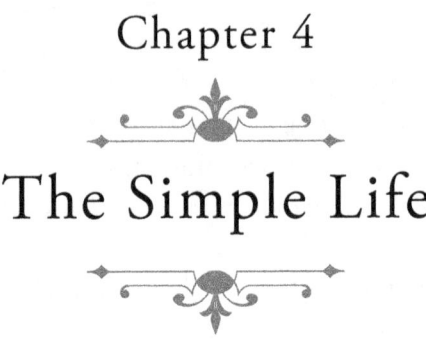

The Simple Life

H ERE IN THE United States of America, we take for granted the concept of owning things. Not just things, but a vast accumulation. Not just *one* thing, but an incredible number of many, *many* things. Just look at the number of garage sales in any given neighborhood. The garage sale is the method of ridding ourselves of some of this excess. We feel good about how much revenue we brought in through our sale. "Look, Dear… we took in $250 today!"

We overlook how much we paid originally for all this stuff. By the way, many of us have a two-car garage, but we can't fit even one car in it.

Now, how does this happen? It is because manufacturers and retailers utilize large programs of advertising and big discount sales to attract buyers. The most popular word in marketing is "Free!" It is hard to resist. We love something that we can get for nothing, or at a discount. Many retail stores raise the cost of an item, then tag it at a substantial discount to make customers think they are getting a bargain.

Another motive – a very important one that makes us buy – is we want to provide things (bicycles, toys, games) for our children and items for our spouse. Americans love to be generous and to be good providers. Also, we like the idea of showing off our new car (if we have one).

Thus, we build up a great inventory of things in the home.

The truth is that nowhere but in places like America does this kind of wealth occur. These are the blessings of capitalism, free enterprise, and liberty.

Let's approach the aspect of complexity in our lives and how we might introduce some simplicity. This would bring a degree of quiet and peace… those welcome visitors in our daily routine. We could remove clutter and give ourselves more space, to tidy up our desk or closet. This suggestion is designed to reduce unnecessary build-up of possessions. Here it is: Buy on the basis of *need* rather than according to urge or impulse.

A major factor in what may be called "the good life" is the very significant concept of being grateful. Gratitude is the quality of being thankful. You can ask, "Am I grateful about anything?" I think that it relates to where a person is **today,** in relation to where she was in the past.

We do much comparison in our lives. We compare people, cars, restaurants, jobs, houses---and much more. One may say, "The present is pretty bad. In the good old days, we had it much better. Kids respected their elders." And then, some people live entirely in the future. "When I get a better position, things will be different." Or, "When we move to a better house, we will be happy."

The truth is: *The present is all you have.* The past is gone forever. The past is a place you can study and learn from. You can see the mistakes that were made and make corrections.

The future is for dream-making – lay out your plans. Nothing wrong with that. But don't live in the past or the future. LIVE FOR THIS DAY. This is what you have. **Today.** Put all your effort and energy in today. *Embrace it.* It is right here for you. Focus on the present. Did you get enough to eat today? Do you have a place to sleep? Do you have clean clothes? Appreciate the gifts that you have this very day.

The Optimist

There are times when things don't go right. I do not think that I am surprising anyone with that statement. The intrinsic nature of life is that occasionally, there will be difficulty, trauma, and sadness. And there will be joy and prosperity and pleasure as well.

The thing you can rely on forever is that *change will happen.* As the Bible says, *It came to pass.* This is basic to growth. We cannot stay the same forever. We need to grow as we need to breathe.

In a situation in which things go from challenging or difficult to unbearable, everything seems to get worse before it gets better. And it isn't just one thing, it is several things happening all at once. This, then, is the place where growth occurs. It may sound totally ridiculous, but this "bad" situation is where we should thank the Universe for the experience. It could take a long time, but you will look back and say, "That was for my highest good. It was a blessing."

To alleviate the feelings of disappointment, we need to adjust our thinking. This is about the most difficult thing in the world to do. But remember... THE THOUGHTS YOU CHOOSE DETERMINE THE EXPERIENCES YOU GET.

Winston Churchill said, "A pessimist sees the difficulty in every opportunity; an optimist sees the opportunity in every difficulty."

If you can choose optimistic thoughts, it is probable you will have some positive outcomes. Just think: You could be an optimist!

Living Free

Living free means freedom from anxiety, fear, doubt, and pain. I am not saying that there will never be pain. That is beyond reality. I am suggesting that we can influence our lifestyle – the things that happen to us.

Take forgiveness, for example. I mentioned this before... forgiving others is one of the keys to living free. One may not be able to forget some offense or annoyance, but forgiveness can happen regardless.

On our journey in life, we eventually come to the realization that what we experience is not about others hurting or offending us. It is clearly about our emotions and how they affect so much of what we do. Our emotions determine how we act, day in and day out. We need to look for the good; it is an inward journey... and the adventure of a lifetime.

What are the blessings you have in your life? A working body, healthy and vital... doing the job you are responsible for and providing a service or product others need? Perhaps it is a comfortable place that you call home? Do you have loving relationships, and leisure time to give balance to your life? And a strength in your spirit to enjoy prosperity and to survive the difficult times? Lastly, have you enough things in your life that contribute to a sense of gratitude and appreciation?

Living free is not free. It means making an effort. Going to school, being on time, observing the rules, maintaining an acceptable attitude within the framework of society's expectations. Achieving a job or position that provides a paycheck to pay rent or mortgage, food, clothing, and supplies for living. At times, getting a job is easier than *keeping* the job.

Over time, there may be a supervisor that you don't get along with or who expects you to do better or work differently. Or he may have personal problems and vents his frustrations on his employees. There are innumerable reasons that employees don't last on the job. According to the Bureau of Labor Statistics, the median length of time that wage and salary workers have worked for their current employer is about 4 years.

Employers are reluctant to hire people who have changed jobs too frequently. Changing positions can suggest a lack of reliability. But staying in the same job when you feel underpaid or underappreciated, can be devastating. Think carefully on securing work. And while on the job, give it your best shot!

Belief

What is belief? It is a mental state. One embraces a concept that he or she utterly knows to be true. It is beyond doubt. For instance, I absolutely know that the earth is round, not flat.

For thousands of years, people believed that the earth was flat. Then, through the ancient Greeks (Pythagoras), it was discovered that our earth was indeed round. As recent as 500 years ago, many still believed it was flat. But Columbus knew better in 1492 when he sailed from Europe to what he thought was India. He simply sought a shorter route.

Beliefs are usually developed over time… and strong feelings of people give depth to belief, with the factor of experience making its contribution. Another factor is wide acceptance. Example: many people now believe in global warming as a significant change in climate systems in the world. This occurred mainly because of government discussion, politics, and media coverage.

Ask an individual about his beliefs and you will learn a great deal about him, *probably more than you need to know!*

The Treasure of Good Health

The person who has good health has a pot of gold but may not realize it. They take it for granted. And the person who has lost it would give just about anything to get it back.

In this section, we will discuss the basic theme of this book – the subject of health. Our physical health is our treasure despite the sacred belief that we are first and foremost *spirit.* The spirit is the nonphysical part of a person; the seat of emotions and character; the soul.

Spirit is the essence of life and the existence of a person; their consciousness; the innate ability to determine their being. Humans seek harmony between the body and the spirit. They are two different entities yet the same, because they form our being… our self.

Let's talk about physical health. Physical health is a reflection of our mental state. What we think and what we believe, (what is in our heart) forms who we are. It determines how we live.

A Plan of Attack. If there is a threat or perceived danger, action to defend such danger will be taken. If an individual is experiencing anger, irritation, or resentment, that is just as real as any threat to our welfare. We need to have a plan of attack.

Now here comes the fork in the road. We have two choices, person *A* or person *B*. Let me explain. Within a person, in the deep and highly personal internal nature of each of us, is a consciousness of acceptance and appreciation, of faith in the friendliness of the universe, of connection with other beings and an attitude that says, life will be better soon. This is a description of *Type A*. This kind of person is generally positive, focusing on forgiveness, health, wealth, and his blessings.

Then there is the flipside of the coin. This person chooses to have a consciousness of antagonism, of resistance, of resentment toward people who criticize him, of belligerence, suspicion, and disunion. That is a description of *Type B*.

We either attract or repel. We build up or tear down. In our thinking, we are positive or negative. So, think of the thoughts you have had today. How many were positive? How many were negative? And apply percentages. My experiment resulted in 70% positive thoughts, and 30% negative thoughts. I am sure there are days when my mood brings 80% negative thoughts, and only 20% positive. With practice, it can be achieved. I say, *Type A* thinkers are winners!

The Human Brain. The brain is the body's control center. Researchers have learned more about the brain in the past decade than they did in the previous one hundred years. The brain contains about 100 billion nerve cells, which communicate with each other at a rate of approximately 200 miles an hour. This data might answer why we have thousands of thoughts every day. The subject of health is extremely interesting, and even exciting because good health is precious to every one of us.

There is another factor – a very significant one – that is involved in good health, and that is one's *mental outlook*.

Heart trouble, stomach ulcers, skin disorders, digestive problems, and many other physical troubles have been traced to a mental origin. What we are saying here is that one's mind is the determining agent that sets in motion the quality of life for the individual.

What a person thinks determines his life! This is not new. This information has been around a very long time.

In this book, we will revisit the subject of health many times. As people grow older, their health may change. In fact, it usually does, bringing on some ills. It is vital for seniors to have good eating habits… choosing what they eat with care. Also, to exercise or go walking or swimming. Getting proper rest is important, of course.

Let's discuss some basic understandings. Philosophers of the past and present have taught concepts, which help to free us from the consequences of disease. These concepts support a belief in *Cause and Effect*. A spiritual man, embracing eternal truths, trusts in the perfection of his body. This requires a deep intelligence… an awareness of human beings as both spirit and body. He understands that healing occurs continually, and that life demands myriad experiences to help us grow spiritually.

Our goal is to be in perfect health: physically, mentally, emotionally, and spiritually. We are forever subject to *change*… and the challenges it presents. They help us to grow. Deepak Chopra says that we have an inner core of being: "a field of non-change that creates personality, ego, and body."

"In order to stay alive," Chopra says, "your body must live on the wings of change. Your stomach, liver, heart, lungs, and brain are being replaced quickly and endlessly. The skin replaces itself once a month; the stomach lining every five days; the liver every six weeks; the skeleton every three months."

I highly recommend *Ageless Body, Timeless Mind,* by Deepak Chopra, M.D., (1993). He is an excellent writer and shares his wisdom of healing. Other Chopra books include *Creating Health, Quantum Healing,* and *Perfect Health.*

To find all of the answers to the questions we pose in the collective human race is, after all, impossible. But we nevertheless keep at it. Age-old wonders about creation, nature, the Infinite, reincarnation, the Universe, and the purpose of life, will continue. ~

Guarding Bob Hope

When I was stationed at Fort Douglas, Utah, Bob Hope and Bing Crosby played a golf tournament to entertain thousands of troops there. To be sure of his safety, ten of us were assigned to form a circle around Bob.

He and Bing were extremely funny and entertaining. What a thrill… to see these two great performers in person. It was a privilege to be in their company.

After the tournament, Bob and his wife, Dolores, visited the local hospital off the base. It was late at night when we escorted the tired couple to their hotel, after a long day.~

Chapter 5

Habits and Life Patterns

WHEN HUMAN BEINGS Are Late. What are some things people are late for? Going to work; lunch with a friend; school; a business meeting; sports practice; going on a date, dropping a child at daycare, a golf game; a seminar or conference; going to movie; a birthday party; a concert.

There are exceptions like traffic or some emergency. But most people are late for things because they do not want to attend the event or keep the commitment they agreed to. The consequences are too great for opposing your partner's wishes, or your boss' demands. Another factor in chronic tardiness is that it is basically a habit. Remember that about 90% of all our behaviors are habits.

Another aspect about being late is this: As this person is heading for the workplace, they speed their vehicle because they think they can make up the time on the road. Now as they come into the office, they have a mixed facial expression of hurry, anxiousness, and guilt. What this does is set their day to be one of tension and nervousness.

You want to have a fun day? Deliberately be early. Walk in with a big smile, greet everyone as if you just won the lottery, and see what kind of day you have.

Science, Belief, and Healing

By studying writers in the field of health and healing, we find that the way people think dramatically influences their health and the process of recovery. More advanced studies in the field of medicine involve the *mental attitude* of patients. Doctors today realize that how the patient views her situation is as important as the diagnosis itself.

In past centuries, it was understood that humans grow old, lose youthful vigor, become senile, and eventually succumb. These ideas, which developed over time, were proposed by parents, teachers, health professionals, and society. They lead us to accept our inevitable fate. *But some refuse to believe it.*

Centenarians---people who are over 100 years old---are increasing in our country; there are over 53,000 centenarians in the United States!

The mind is a vital aspect of aging in the individual. Deepak Chopra states that, "Aging is changeable; it can speed up, slow down, stop for a time, even reverse itself." A positive belief about recovering one's health is essential in maintaining a life of continued energy and enthusiasm.

I have always believed that when an individual has some kind of connection to a Higher Being, (Source, Universal Intelligence, Father, or God) that such person enjoys life more. He has a feeling or guidance... a deep-seated humility that recognizes an awareness of spirituality. He has strength and confidence in the earth experience. I believe that within each of us there is a treasure; a presence of the Divine; the subconscious; an intuition or intelligence.

I suspect that it doesn't work with every person, though there is validity in the concept. But with time, it is likely to be embraced by the individual.

We all have our opinions about a Creator and our beginnings... the age-old mysteries of life. We ask questions like, "Why is there so much suffering in the world?" This freedom of thought is a gift... the gift of *free will*. We are not robots; we have choices to make. What to do; how to be; what to think. It is up to us.

The mysteries of life. Now about the spiritual... I don't believe in a god up in the sky, nor in a man-god with a long white beard; a human-type being who punishes the "bad," and awards the "good." I believe Spirit is the best of the unseen: love, kindness, generosity, humility, guilelessness; that we are here to learn through many lives... *eternal* life; that we are unable to define the Divine except in human terms.

I believe that our Universe operates in an Intelligence beyond any human comprehension; that Nature and Universal Law set the events of our world in motion for our experience and growth, but not necessarily for our understanding. Not with any presumption but with enduring humility do I attempt this description... yet stated with a deep heart and recognizing that every human being sets his beliefs as he feels.

National Public Radio presented the outstanding series, *Downton Abbey*, by Julian Fellowes – all about early 20th Century Royalty. There is a scene in which one of the characters says, "What are we here for?" The answer is given: "To get through life as best we can."

There are so many people in the world that seem to just be getting by, not with much energy or enthusiasm or pleasure. We can look at that differently. It could be just an episode in their life story... something they are going through, and things could change so that a better situation is soon to occur.

Then there are those who have the drive and ambition to improve themselves, through trade school, education, hobbies, reading, and the like. Each individual makes choices that determines their lifestyle. What are we here for? *I do not think it is to merely get through life as best we can.*

Let us use this example: With 20-30 delicious choices you have at a Swedish smorgasbord, you gladly choose the foods that are appealing to you. This is true with jobs, schools, relationships, vehicles, stores, apartments, electronics, houses, clothing, auto mechanics, and hair stylists. But the person who makes no choice has *also* made a choice! Decide what you want – make a plan, rather than let circumstances dictate your fate.

Of Wisdom

When I was planning this book and choosing a title, I thought about my readers. I wanted to bring a substantial offering of wisdom to my reader. "How do I do this?" I asked myself. "Am I a wise person?" An interesting question, and difficult to answer.

I am continually seeking ways to better myself. The way I attempt to solve this is to read and learn all I can. Gaining wisdom takes time and a lot of patience. I have been at it my entire life, and I thoroughly enjoy this journey.

The following discussion is about *The Seasons of Life,* a piece written by Dr. Michael Gott of Houston, Texas. "Everything is temporary" says Gott. "Spirit is moving in and out of form." I think this means that every life, every event, everything in its essence, is in some way connected to a Higher Being or Intelligence; *Spirit*. Every item exists because of some energy, force, or reason... the understanding of which is beyond human comprehension.

Do we have any control over the events in our lives? I submit that, to an extent, we do. I am not sure we can control how long we will live. But I believe an individual influences his or her length of stay by many aspects, one of which is the depth of her determination. In other words, our desire and belief.

Here is another thing. The decision to live long usually is joined with other traits such as love and happiness, kindness, patience, generosity, humility, good-temperedness, courtesy, unselfishness, guilelessness, and sincerity. What I'm suggesting is this: If you want to live a deeply joyful, harmonious loving life, this is certainly possible but it is going to take some effort.

The natural impact of one's emotions comes into play--- constantly. So get into the habit of accepting a situation rather than criticizing or arguing. Consider discussion rather than altercation. Be thoughtful of another's feelings. This is not easy, but it is well worth the effort.

With human relations, we are either attracting people to us or we are driving them away. The essence of human relations is treating others in such a way that they desire your company and are sad when you go. Let them say, "Can't you stay a little longer?"

"There are three rules for getting along with others," said Henry James, father of psychology, "*Rule 1*: Be kind. *Rule 2*: Be kind. And *Rule 3*: Be kind."

Do you want to make people like you? I have one rule: Smile big and look into their eyes.

The Universe

<u>A Mini Course In Astronomy</u>. What is this about? I will explain. This incredible place – this Universe – is our home. When we talk about astronomy... the vastness, motion, speed, and nature... we learn more about our humanity. Humans tend to see themselves as larger than life. But looking at the stars is humbling. We learn that our earth is actually quite small. Our sun, a medium-sized star, is a *million* times bigger than the earth.

It was the Greeks who first studied the earth and the universe about 300 years B.C. They proved that the earth was a fiery ball, but they thought it was the center of the universe. Ptolemy's theories were widely accepted; they were in harmony with the writings of Aristotle. John Kepler studied the movements of the planets, and the Italian professor, Galileo, made the first practical telescope. For the next 1000 years or more, scientists (Polish astronomer Copernicus, Englishman Sir Isaac Newton, Danish astronomer Tycho Brahe and others) contributed to the study of the universe.

Modern astronomers know that humans can survive on earth because the sun is precisely positioned so that we don't freeze or burn up.

Scientists have proven that the universe is actually expanding, minute by minute. Ninety-nine percent of the universe is invisible to people on our tiny planet. How fast is it expanding? Certain nearby galaxies and clusters of galaxies like those in the constellation Virgo expand at a rate of <u>750 miles per second</u>. That would be 100 times around our earth in one hour. This expansion has been taking place for **billions of years.**

As to the size of the universe, we need to use *the speed of light* to measure distances. Light travels at 186,000 miles per second. Other than our sun, the nearest star to Earth is Alpha Centauri, which is about 4 light years away. Our group of planets and stars form the *Milky Way*. There are over 100 billion stars in our galaxy. And there are <u>millions</u> of galaxies in the known universe.

When I look up at the stars and think about the universe, it makes my problems appear very small.

Some theorists speculate that there are planets in the universe which can sustain human life. So, does this mean that we will be able to vacation to other planets? It certainly is a possibility!

My Talk With God

I have always found that Spirit is available. I wanted to know if my lifestyle was appropriate for good health and a long life. So, I requested a talk with Spirit and posed my question.

Spirit asked, "Do you sleep 7-8 hours per night?"
"Yes, Spirit. I do" I replied.
'That's good. Do you eat breakfast every day?"
"Yes, Sir."
Spirit continued, "Do you eat between meals?"
"Uh---well, yes."
"Hmm. Is your weight normal? Not more than 10%-20% overweight?"
"I am okay there, Lord."
"Let's talk about exercise. Do you do sports, work out, go on walks, garden or swim?"
"I play table tennis, Spirit."
"Do you smoke or drink?"
"No, Spirit... none of that."

God indicated that if one does 2-3 healthy habits, they might live 25 extra years; if they do 6-7 healthy habits, they might live 35 extra years. Spirit finished by saying, "Your body sends unmistakable messages whenever its needs aren't being met. Millions of electrical impulses are coursing through the heart and brain all day, every day. Be sure you attend to your body!"

I thanked Spirit, not only for the information, but for the many blessings I have received. Our talk concluded with me smiling from ear to ear. ~

Chapter 6

Some Secrets About Health

O UR BODY IS the product of our thoughts. In 2006, quantum physicist Dr. John Hagelin stated, "In medical science, we are beginning to understand the degree to which thoughts and emotions actually determine the function of our bodies."

Modern medicine involves the mind, feelings, and emotions---as well as the body. An individual opens himself to feel wonder and joy, and all the great things that the universe has in store for him. These include good health and abundance. But when you have negative thoughts, you will feel the aches and pains life can bring. It is a major life decision, requiring an individual to discard influences laid upon him as a child; the programming we may have received, and the fearful impulses set into our psyche.

Actually, the decision to live your life in a positive way requires tremendous concentration *daily* or perhaps many times a day, taking strong mental action and thinking with determination. When someone offends you, or when you think you weren't treated right, that is the moment to take action; to fight the ego. Find a way to counter the negativity. Here's a good tip: Ask, "How did I contribute to this problem?"

I can't tell you how important it is to choose good thoughts. Be kind, polite, and generous. It will open the door to miracles.

Most people have stress in their lives. They are nervous about their work or concerned about their partner or children. They are dismayed that they don't get along with their in-laws. Most of the time, we take ourselves too seriously. With this in mind, let's look at how an overworked person at their desk with many responsibilities responds when you call.

You've been on hold for a while and may not feel kindly toward this person. But you can brighten their day. You might start off by saying, "Oh, good morning. Could you please help me?" That doesn't take much effort at all.

What is happening here is this: you are being polite and thoughtful of another. Your voice is gentle, not terse or demanding. You will receive the help you need and at the same time, you are letting them know you appreciate them. You are kind; you say "thank you." After all, customer service is not easy.

I use this technique a lot. I have fun with it; sometimes I make her laugh. It is like a release of pressure, and lifts both giver and receiver.

The Meaning of Life

If you ask a few people, "What is the meaning of life?" you will probably get answers that are very different. One person may say, "It is painful and constantly disappointing. If I plan something, I can count on it going sour." Another might say, "The beauty and pleasure of this life is joyful."

I found a section in the third volume of *God Given, Answers To Your Questions,* (Denise Bennett, Ph.D.), that gives exceptional answers to this question. Let me quote part of this offering:

> *The life is a mirror, as you know. Every belief you hold about the meaning of life---the meaning of all things for that matter---reveals what your particular lesson is at a given moment. If a brother says that life is a spiritual journey and its purpose is to know Self, then that is exactly what he is learning. And if your brother says that life has no meaning at all, with a bitterness in his tone, then you know his lesson is forgiveness.*

> *It is really quite simple. As you develop your awareness and grow in wisdom, your answer will change. What you believed yesterday is not what you believe today, nor is it what you will believe tomorrow.*

The nature of the experiences we have had paints a picture based on happy or unpleasant events. We need to grow in wisdom, to be careful in our choices, and to guide others and ourselves in the best way--- because we have the power to do so.

What's the Difference?

What is the difference between *thinking* and *feeling*? There is a vast difference. Thinking is the process of using one's mind to contemplate and consider what we view as important in our life. It is not something that one is flippant about; it is usually significant. An individual weighs evidence or factual indications and uses his rational judgment in making his decisions.

Where thinking is direct, organized, and structured, feeling can be embracing, nurturing, subtle, or even ethereal. While thinking is more from the surface, feeling taps into something deeper, which is vitally important. When you shop for a new vehicle in the showroom, much of the decision relates to color, styling, that new car smell, and how it **feels** to sit behind the wheel.

As minister, Dr. Jesse Jennings (Houston, Texas) stated, "Thinking may steer, but feeling propels."

Reality and Imagination

Let's consider two areas of thinking: **reality** and **imagination**. You will recall that we have thousands of thoughts every day. This occurs day and night, 24 hours a day. Think about the times you awaken from sleep, and you recall a dream you had. Maybe you laugh because it was silly, or perhaps it frightened you... like falling from a high place. These thoughts may come from the imagination. We call them dreams.

Sometimes thoughts develop into ideas. You think of something that you need to work out or improve on. As you begin to sleep, think deeply about the problem and maybe you will wake up with a solution.

Each experience that we have starts with an idea that is created by the mind. The activities we enjoy – they all began as an idea in our mind. Our conscious mind is always creating. If we accept these ideas, they become form, which means reality.

As an 8-year-old, I dreamed of being an airline pilot. I drew airplanes; I pretended to fly. Eventually, I became a pilot at age 50. I attended ground school, took flying lessons, and learned to fly the Cessna 150 and the Cessna 172, (private planes). I enjoyed this great hobby for 12 years.

The point is, my mind accepted the idea, and the idea became reality.

Now, reality is the state of being real; the totality of real things… things that *really exist,* not just ideals of them. But, reality cannot be determined without perception. Perception is what people hear, see, and think based on their beliefs.

Here's what the publication *Elite Daily* says about people's perceptions:

> *The way people view you and the way you present yourself is the impression you will leave behind. As you go about the business of carrying out your life, people will make judgments about your appearance, personality, and capabilities. If you don't like the way your life is playing out, you can always take charge of your own perception of reality. You are in control of your story.*

The Gift of Health

Here are some authors I've enjoyed over the years, which I sought answers to questions I have had. Like most of us, I have wondered about pain and suffering, the universe, eternity, the meaning of life... God, Spirit, the soul, the beginning of time... about parents and children, love, wealth, and the gift of health.

Frederick Bailes	Ralph Waldo Emerson
Raymond Charles Barker	Louise Hay
Eric Butterworth	Napoleon Hill
H. Emilie Cady	Ernest Holmes
Dale Carnegie	Norman Vincent Peale
Deepak Chopra	Catherine Ponder
Henry Drummond	Florence Scovel Shinn
Wayne W. Dyer	Susan Smith Jones
Mary Baker Eddy	Thomas Troward

In all this reading, I found the path to be very fascinating and even exciting at times. I have had good discussions with family and friends about health, philosophy, education, and religion.

In this section, I will share my beliefs about **good health.** It is a recurring theme throughout this book and has great importance to me... and hopefully, to you as well.

We are given the gift of good health, many of us. When we experience sickness, it can be a way to deal with fears and anxieties, anger, jealousy, frustration, etc. These thoughts are toxic and affect our health. We work hard to achieve happiness... to gain stability and success... to find love. Why is it so difficult to achieve these things?

Much of the problem is the damage done by emotional stress. Our emotions are a basic part of life; no way around it. We are apt to choose negative neural circuits when someone offends or disappoints us; when we don't like the answer a person gives us.

In addition, the impressions we received as children – the things we learned from parents, teachers and others – has a large influence as to how we now react to the actions of others.

When television ads or healthcare professionals or insurance companies try to inform and provide products or services to the public, these words and images may cause us to develop a fear-consciousness in the mind. This can happen without our awareness and the damage may remain for a lifetime.

For some persons, these impressions build fear that affects the body day and night. Multiply this by many, many situations, such as an abusive parent or relative that instills fear in a child. This might establish a lifelong pattern of apprehension.

Illness, then, is often a basic sign of stress, fear, or emotional disturbance. If one can remove these blocks, people could have a life of good health… and the treasure they long for. ~

How to Get Out of Guard Duty

I was stationed at Daejon, South Korea for a year, basically on the task of guard duty. The war had been over for nearly three months, but the Japanese were trained to die for their country and emperor rather than surrender. The concept of surrendering was eternal shame. On guard duty, it was not unusual to hear rifle shots fired.

Daejon had a new military installation. Quonset huts were built for housing, recreation, and Post Exchange where men could buy toiletries, cigarettes, soft drinks, etc. Also in process was a military airstrip.

It was Sunday and I was off duty. I saw the Commanding Officer, Captain Davis, walking toward me. I brought up a sharp military salute. The C.O. returned the salute. Then, he said, "Soldier!" Uh, oh. I turned around and approached the Captain. He said, "What's your name, Soldier?" "Private Wiesel, Sir." I answered. Then he said, "Private, how would you like to work in the P.X.?"

I said, "Anything to get off guard duty, Sir." I think the Captain liked my honesty. I had a new job! I was to report to the P.X Quonset hut the very next day.

Chapter 7

Healing, Feeling, and the Mind

T HE WAY WE feel about ourselves is a vital component in the happiness equation. Our self-image develops over time between infancy and childhood; it is a combination of ego, personality, and memory functioning, and involves our social connections with others. Yet, we humans are unique… completely different and separate from every other person.

The world is divided into reality and illusion, but what we see in our surroundings is *us*. In more familiar terms, **perception is reality.** This is so important for healing. One person says, "I see her getting well quickly. I am certain she will heal and be better very soon." Another person says, "She looks terrible. I doubt she will recover. Most people do very poorly from that circumstance."

It is similar to the way people greet the new day. The optimist says, "Good morning, God!" The pessimist says, "Good God, it's morning!"

Biochemical research was done isolating brain chemicals… specifically, serotonin, a pleasure chemical. A person who is high in serotonin is one who feels a sense of well-being; an individual with low serotonin frequently is depressed, discouraged, or ill-tempered.

One person enjoys a good feeling about life; he feels love in the world. He can recover more quickly from the challenges, disappointments, and diseases that may occur, than one who is basically fed up and negative about life.

Mother Mary Teresa was a Catholic nun. She was beloved, especially in India, where she spent most of her life. People who observed her work with children were tested. Just by watching Mother Teresa, there were chemical indications of increased immunity levels for those observers.

A research project took place at Duke University involving people who had recent surgery. Half of this group were prayed for and half were not. The results were amazing. Persons who were prayed for, healed faster. This shows the power of prayer, and the way healing can be affected. I don't think God needs our prayers; I think *we* need our prayers.

When you pray for someone, two things happen: *1)* You feel better, and *2)* possibly *they* feel better.

I believe that we have the choice of being everything we care to be… that within each of us, there is good and evil; love and hate. We are a combination of opposites. It is not enough for a person to speak nicely or think positively. Sorry, that is not reality; that is fantasy. We must back our words with action. From the Bible: "Faith without works is dead."

I do think that we are Spirit and flesh at the same time. To reach authenticity, I face myself. I am the first to admit my faults. Yes, I *could be better*, but that's an uphill road. If I want to go there, I am going to have to work hard.

If I want to be loving, I need to be selfless, and sensitive to others. That's another difficult task. "Life is hard work," many have said. Our decisions are personal actions or perhaps *reactions*, as we deal with our complex lives. Things began to form: beliefs, fears, love, affection---the whole personality, and it formed early on. This is the child, wanting to be protected; the adolescent yearning to be accepted; the adult wanting to find a mate; the older person seeking love and companionship.

We have the freedom to think, act, and feel. We are able to make choices – life-changing decisions – throughout our life. At any time, we can replace anger, distrust, and bitterness with forgiveness, love, and compassion. It is clear that the physical, mental, and emotional health systems of an individual rely entirely on the way we apply behavioral patterns.

My son gave me the gift of an excellent book: *The Path To Love*, by Deepak Chopra. It offers a comprehensive guideline for human relationships. Originally published in 1973, this bestseller defines the power of Spirit in one's life. I highly recommend it.

The situations and events we encounter relate to our feelings about them. The way we look at our job, relationships, neighbors, relatives---in other words, our judgment---is going to impact perception and create our feelings about them. Here's a secret: when a person makes peace with his present situation, he is set free. A door has opened. And then, there could be an opportunity for a much happier situation.

Maybe we cannot change all the circumstances of our lives, but we can change how we feel about them, and this might bring about a sense of well-being and peace of mind.

One of my all-time favorite films is Frank Capra's *It's a Wonderful Life* (1947) starring Jimmy Stewart and Donna

Reed, along with a great supporting cast. Stewart's character is George Bailey, who lives in a small town. The film explores the pain of normal life as well as the joy. Devastating circumstances drive George to consider suicide, and that's when he meets Clarence, his guardian angel.

Clarence views the events in George's life, then comments that "each man's life touches so many other lives." He helps George to see the value in all he has endured.

While each of our lives vary in qualitative and quantitative ways, there is the basic nature of life: the experience of pain and suffering. The purpose of pain is to help us learn and grow. Then lessons, well-learned and absorbed, blossom for beauty in our soul.

From *Emmanuel's Book,* compiled by Pat Rodegast and Judith Stanton, I offer this passage that may provide some insight into why we have pain.

Be comforted and walk your life in Light and trust, for nothing will come to you that is not meant to be. There is nothing that can happen in your life that in any way threatens your soul. Indeed, all of life experience enhances its awareness. There is nothing that does not serve the process of your soul's growth.

A Little Affirmation For You

What is an affirmation? I will tell you. It is the practice of positive thinking. It is the belief that you can achieve success in life. It is a feeling that you have some control in your life. As a matter of fact, it attests to your desire to reprogram your thinking; actually, you are going to reprogram your *subconscious mind.*

Here is the process: You send a brief, specific message. You make a statement and repeat it many, many times. You do this to get results. Believe in yourself; you can do it. Never give up. *Never.* Set a time, say 5 minutes daily. **Every day.** Try a month, then two months. Be the power that you are. What is your message or goal? Money? Health? Relationship? Promotion? And then be consistent.

If you are not going to be consistent – if you affirm one day and then skip a week, you're bound to fail. You must make it a habit. Be brief---just a simple phrase. Start with, "I am...." But do not use negatives. Do not say, "I'm not poor..." The subconscious omits "not"_and hears "I'm poor." Instead, say, "I am rich!"

Did you know that repetition is the mother of all learning? Here is an affirmation I've repeated again and again...

I am in perfect health. I am in perfect health. I am in perfect health!

<u>Hollywood Actress Used Declarations</u>. Olivia De Havilland (1916 – 2020) was nominated five times for best actress, winning twice for *The Heiress* and *To Each His Own*. She enjoyed a long career in Hollywood, acting in many fine pictures, and her best-known film, *Gone With the Wind*. She lived in Paris with her husband for several decades. On July 1, 2006, when she turned 90 years of age, she declared that she would live to be 100. *She lived to be 104.* She said that **love, laughter, and learning** was the secret to a happy life.

You *Can* Take It With You

In Earth time, we have seconds, minutes, hours, days, weeks, and so on. Eternity is very different. In fact, there is no time. Now, while you are here on Earth, you have probably worked hard and collected things. Perhaps you have a savings account. Maybe you have a house, cars, even a boat or other possessions. Let's say you have an estate. You've probably heard the expression, "You can't take it with you." Well, I say, you *can!* Here's how: In the years left, each day, bless your money and all you have in your life. The things, the people you love, those who love you, your spouse and family, close friends, your pets, perhaps your neighbors, and even the tax collector.

WHAT WAS THAT? Did you say your tax collector?? Are you nuts? Who wrote this book?

Okay, calm down. I can explain…

Yes, I said tax collector. Now, let me be very clear. I want you to *bless the money, the things, the people you love, those who love you, your neighbors, friends, pets-----and EVERYTHING.* Bless the food, the clean water you drink, your health, and your loving companion.

What is a blessing? It is a prayer, asking for God's protection. Blessings have to do with gratitude and approval; your acceptance of something or someone in your life. A blessed event brings pleasure, contentment, or good fortune. I want those things… *I want pleasure, contentment, and good fortune.*

It relates to the concept of "what goes around, comes around." It's decision time. I submit to you that we have here, in this universe, incredible abundance… things, yes, and also love and caring and affection, and giving to others. If you accept this way of life, what will be the results? Better health? Greater prosperity? A more peaceful, joyful life? There are no guarantees, but your positive outlook is a good start.

You take it with you when you embrace every moment of this life experience; you caress all that is, dismiss the negative, and open your heart to give *and receive* the best for the time you have here.

That is filling your soul with divine memories... and taking it with you.

The Nature of Human Beings

<u>Hate.</u> Now we get to an uncomfortable discussion. It is this: hate is a common emotion in most people. I don't want to believe it but recognize that it is valid. Sigmund Freud believed that our instincts drive much of our behavior; they can be hateful and destructive. He said that love is oftentimes mixed with hate.

Some modern psychiatrists say that even loving adults seem to need something to despise, like doing some difficult or unpleasant task. Researchers found that babies become agitated when they do not receive attention to their needs. But hate – anger – can have the function of moving humans to act. Frustration gets the personality going. It may be the reason that ambition forms in people.

History reveals that governments have been overthrown; dictators have come to power by creating paranoia and hate in the people; acts inducing war, threat from other countries, and a general uprising against the norm, moving to extreme emotionality that fosters rebellion.

Jung felt that people should make an honest inspection of their behavior, facing their emotions and adjust accordingly where possible. I recognize that behavior is <u>caused.</u> A person builds animosity or hate when they feel attacked. He carries that anger for a long time. Then, maturity may bring an attitude adjustment. But some individuals carry anger and hate all of their lives; such anger frequently turns to violence.

Do you think watching violence on television (games or movies) releases more of the same in us? I have always believed that watching violence stimulates violence.

Fortunately, there is evidence that every human being has some goodness in him and a healthy conscience which, with society's enduring encouragement, allows us to achieve a level of civility, enabling society to survive.

Fear. During World War II, German aircraft flew over a London bomb shelter, and a bomb struck nearby. The lights went out. Not a sound was heard. The terrified souls inside died, not by the bomb but by fear... tremendous fear *alone*, killed all 200 people in the shelter.

Fear can control an entire nation. In the midst of a paralyzing depression in our nation, President Roosevelt said, "The only thing we have to fear is fear itself."

Being afraid is a valuable part of our system, designed to protect us when danger is present. Other fears reveal our personality and beliefs. There is fear of death, fear of aging, fear of guns, fear of animals, and fear of heights, to name just a few.

Mostly, our fears are *conditioned responses*... deep influences based on our experiences. Fear, then, has important functioning for the human. But some people are always afraid. They dread losing their job, their relationship, their finances, or their health. They suffer from sleeplessness and worry about persons who might attack them. Fears can be intensified by a negative attitude, criticism, or complaining. Here's an interesting fact: 80% of all fears and anxieties **never happen.**

Mild fears are somewhat different. Humans sometimes enjoy the thrill of exciting amusement park rides like roller coasters and parachute drops to achieve "kicks" and fun. There are activities that satisfy these needs, such as skiing, racing, and mountain climbing. I learned to fly a private plane years ago. I flew almost every weekend; every time I turned on the key and that engine started, my heart pounded with excitement as

I went up in the sky. I suppose that was a "mild" fear, but it felt more like *moderate!*

One interesting type of fear is not being accepted in social situations. This individual seeks validation; he greatly depends on the opinions of others, rather than on self-esteem. When a person relies on the admiration of friends or relatives, his personality is jeopardized. For years, public schools have emphasized the value of a healthy sense of self-worth to deal with the vagaries of life.

Fearful adults feel that the world is too difficult or even threatening. They may have been traumatized. Many people *feel the fear and do it anyway.* (Take a look at Susan Jeffer's book with this title) They go about their business, doing the things that need to be done… and function with strength, purpose and integrity that is the mainstay of society.

Anger. This very common human emotion is everywhere. We release anger as a safety valve---to blow off steam. This is usually a healthy act. When we get angry and think about it later, we sometimes have regrets; we are surprised that we lost our temper.

It is a commonly held belief that to suppress anger is definitely not smart. Yet when we lose our temper, we are filled with remorse. We want to believe that we are civilized and understanding and mature, and then without warning, we lose our calm; we experience self-disappointment.

Psychologists say that anger is the least civilized attribute of man. Psychiatrist Karl Menninger wrote that "the human child begins his life in anger."

Studies of adult anger indicate that we lose our tempers like babies do, mainly because the situation or action that occurred made us feel insecure or helpless, weak, or powerless.

Adults are most irritable when they are ill or tired, or when they are hungry. When they lose their temper, they show it by loudness, profanity, or perhaps hitting something. They will let off steam for ten minutes. This is followed by moodiness for some length, perhaps days or longer.

Happily, most mature individuals do not experience temper tantrums or violence. Much of the time, disturbing behaviors relate to people who have experienced abuse, exploitation, or other aberrant treatment. They tend to carry hurt feelings for a long time. Perhaps these feelings occurred at a young age. Hostility and anger may cause rejection or disapproval from others, and this manifests more anger.

A male adult with a short fuse may have had a mother who was indifferent or insensitive. In her book entitled, "The Fears Men Live By," Selma G. Hirsh comments, "It was startling to see how often the anger expressed by the adult turned out to be nearly as old as he *himself* was."

This data begs the question, "Shouldn't it be vastly important for mothers and fathers to recognize the effect their actions have on their new baby?"

Psychoanalyst Karen Horney, in observing angry people, said, "They tend to demand power and insist on always being right, as they cope with what they see as a hostile world."

In the *Archives of General Psychiatry*, it was reported that people who swallow anger – who are extremely angry, but say nothing and don't talk about their feelings – tend to suffer headaches, ulcers, an increase in blood pressure and skin disorders, as a result of suppressed anger.

Within the family, each child is raised somewhat differently. My parents certainly had their difficulties. I had a rare gift, as my mother and aunt were identical twins. This gave me the happy experience of having two deeply loving and caring mothers. Being a parent is not easy. It is wise to release any anger you hold, knowing they did the best they could.

The Tale of Jumping Mouse

Courage in humans can be remarkable or unremarkable. There are many reasons for the expression of courage. One may be a showy individual who tries something dangerous, longing for recognition. Another may feel guilt or envy, or daringly fearless.

A less obvious courage is the way a person accepts life and its challenges, and accepts himself the way he is… his faults and his mistakes. Courage is his willingness to correct poor behavior, and the way he is respectful of others even though he may disagree with them.

Courage is the ability to love others, and oneself.

The greater courage is that of ordinary human beings, doing the everyday work of living, meeting their responsibilities, and maintaining their strength and integrity. It is a willingness to continue on, despite occasional terrible events and disappointment that may appear in their lives. It is a testimonial to ordinary human beings.

The following story, *The Legend of Jumping Mouse,* tells about how courage can dramatically change one's life. My thanks go to Rev. Sally Robbins, minister in Asheville, North Carolina, for her lovely tale.

He began as an ordinary mouse, scurrying through the prairie grass. But Mouse kept hearing the roar of rushing water, so he left the safety of his home and began his journey. He found the river and met Frog, who advised him to crouch down and then to jump as high as he could. When Mouse jumped, he saw the sacred mountains, and as he descended, he fell into the river.

Crawling out of the river, Mouse was furious that he was all wet. Frog asked, "What did you see when you jumped?" Mouse replied, "I saw the sacred mountains. Frog replied, "You have a new name now. It is Jumping Mouse."

This story about his journey shows that Jumping Mouse can no longer creep as he did before. Now he jumps and leaps. Despite disappointment and fear, his courage brought him to the sacred mountains. ～

Chapter 8

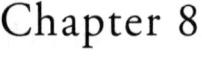

A Bit of Philosophy

D O W E H A V E control of our life? Do we know how long we are going to live? Will we have excellent health in our lifetime? Is there an afterlife?

Scientists, philosophers, and behaviorists study the history of humans and discover great similarities *and differences* in human behavior, as well as varying belief systems. Philosophers such as Ralph Waldo Emerson, Paul Edwards, Raymond Moody, Elisabeth Kuebler-Ross, and Baruch Spinoza indicate a belief in immortality.

Interview a thousand persons and you get a thousand opinions about immortality. In fact, does anyone know the purpose of our existence? Can anyone describe God? I could go on and on with questions. It is a very fascinating and absorbing business.

I recognize that not all men think alike. The beauty in that is the idea that we have free will to choose what our life may be like… *IF* we make the effort that goes along with our dreams.

Ralph Waldo Emerson was one philosopher who felt that a person could believe deeply in the afterlife and have a desire to continue life, and that such event could occur. Who can prove this?

Our composition is body, mind, and soul. The mind, our command center, makes decisions through the *conscious mind*. The soul is our spirit, giving us ability to reason, to think; it is our memory bank.

Let's discuss the body. Essentially, we need to care for the body, subject to all we have learned about it. It is fifty-trillion cells, organs, and thousands of miles of blood vessels. It is a miraculous machine. Of vast significance is what we believe in our heart.

Strong belief creates strong possibilities. A person of strong doubt will close those doors of possibility.

I firmly believe that there are influences in life that propel us to act. A parent insists that the child puts away his toys before coming to dinner; a sixth grader needs to finish her homework before she can play with her friends or watch television; a high-schooler has to meet his responsibilities before he can borrow the car.

At an advanced level, an individual discovers that a raise in pay correlates to his performance; a promotion would depend on superior work. All these activities are designed to bring about success in one's accomplishments with a proud family looking on and celebrating with us.

Ernest Holmes writes, "The ability to control your experiences and have them result in happiness, prosperity and success lies in your own mind and the way you use it." We are really in charge of our own affairs, and the way life comes about. Personally, I feel that the errors and mistakes in life are there for specific reasons; they are there for <u>lessons.</u> If we can accept the situation or event and correct it, then declare that it will not occur again (if possible), then it becomes complete.

Many writers and philosophers have written about the nature of life, the afterlife, and universal concepts such as good and evil. Moody wrote *Life After Life*, a bestseller which describes near-death experiences. Zoroaster discussed monotheistic religions and created *Zoroastriasm*, stating that we have free will. He said that a good life means preserving and perpetuating life, following a useful occupation, and raising a family.

Other writers include Kierkegaard, Beckett... and Descartes, who was a French philosopher. He said the universe is divided between the physical and the spiritual and understood the mind-body connection. He was a brilliant philosopher and far ahead of his time.

Reincarnation: I Enjoyed the Ride, Let's Do It Again

Let us begin with someone named, "Edward." A fair amount of harmony occurred within Edward's life. He enjoyed a nice family, some great friends, a substantial career, excellent health, and a long life. Along with these go pleasures such as a sense of power and purpose in living.

Dear Readers, I have drawn the character of Edward into this discussion to introduce the subject of *Reincarnation.*

Edward is a happy person who is self-aware and believes that life has choices. He wants to live again. With the mistakes Edward made in life, he feels that he learned from each experience. Also, he feels that there are many aspects to reincarnation; that it is a collection of consciousness, perhaps from many persons.

This is another thing Edward learned from a dependable source: if reincarnation exists, one would experience many lives. And that any given lifetime may be completely different from the one before.

For thousands of years, Hindus and Buddhists have held a view of life that says, you are born; you live; you die... and because nobody's perfect, your soul returns again and again until the lessons are learned; until the soul evolves as dictated by the complex plan for each of us.

Ralph Waldo Emerson, American philosopher, introduced thoughts about karma in the early 19th Century. Karma refers to "action," such as the personal actions of humans in dealing with their complex lives, or events that form an endless chain of cause and effect (action and reaction); events that began deep in the past, that formed karmic bonds that bind us together.

Examples: a child, longing to be protected and cared for; an adolescent wanting approval; an adult, desiring to find love. Karma ties us to old desires and future ones simultaneously. If one runs up debt, that debt will be paid; if one has items owed to him, he will be paid back. The universe, in time, settles all.

We offer some basic statements that relate to **reincarnation, karma** and **soul** as drawn from Buddhist and Hindu beliefs...

Every experience of the soul provides eternal lessons.
Choice mostly overrules destiny.
Your soul is the absolute essence of you.
From the body's perspective, the soul is the conscious animating life within it.

Humans are almost always reborn as humans.
The soul exists. All human beings are a combination of
physical body, and immortal soul.
The soul is pure consciousness, pure energy, pure being.
It exists on a timeless non-physical level of reality. It is
Spirit or divine light or love.
All our good and bad karma enters our new body.
All souls are on a mission to evolve through their own
experiences and efforts.
To evolve is to become increasingly self-aware, and
to have a unique expression of Spirit. We evolve most
effectively in physical form.
We become entities with greater and greater levels of
love, power and wisdom.

Evolution of the soul comes about through individual experience and choice. A soul evolves by making choices – big and small – and by experiencing the effects of each. To do so, the soul takes a new body for a lifetime; it experiences being physically limited and separated from others. This is an illusion, because the soul is never limited or separate. But the illusion creates enough desire, fear, and other pressures to cause the individual to experience conflicts and dilemmas and to make choices. These experiences serve as lessons for the soul.

The soul learns that all choices have consequence, not just for the self but for everyone involved. The soul learns best through a "compare and contrast" process. One lifetime is not enough to experience all circumstances for the full spectrum of his evolution. A being may experience both male and female, victim and perpetrator, student and teacher.

Those experiences may include a complete range of possible relationships and lessons, and gradually the soul becomes more self-aware, as more of its true capabilities are revealed.

Let me pose this example where a specific lesson is needed. A prejudiced man is abusive to a black teen-aged girl. In a subsequent life, he becomes a black orphan girl, aged seven, which enables him to experience dramatic concepts in his soul.

Rebirth is one of the foundational doctrines of Buddhism. It refers to actions driven by intention. It is a deed done *deliberately* through body, speech, or mind which leads to future consequences.

While many mainstream scientists reject belief in the soul and other concepts (such as reincarnation and karma), at least a fourth of all Americans believe that the soul evolves through multiple lives.

When people discuss reincarnation, they frequently ask, "Why don't we remember past lives?" Edgar Cayce said, "We do not have to remember; we are the sum total of all our memories. We manifest them in our habits, our idiosyncrasies, our likes and dislikes, our talents, our physical and emotional strengths and vulnerabilities." (From *Edgar Cayce on Reincarnation,* Noel Langley, New York, 1969.)

What Are Your Intentions?

In my day, a father would have a talk with the young man dating his daughter and ask this question. The correct answer would be to marry her, of course.

An intention is an idea that you expect to carry out, or your goal, aim or purpose. Wayne Dyer said that intention is an energy that surrounds us; that we can train ourselves to tune into this energy for our own self-development.

One's intention is a plan. Let us say a person (we will name him Carl) has been on the job for several years but has not been given an opportunity to advance. He has a good work ethic, and he hasn't taken many days off, though the work is uninteresting. Actually, it's rather boring most of the time. Also, the supervisor has criticized this individual, occasionally being rude and abusive.

When there were disagreements, Carl has tried to defend his actions, sometimes just to improve the procedures that might streamline production for the company. This seems to exacerbate the problem, and that's when he stops trying.

That summarizes the background in this situation. Now to affect the change that may be appropriate here requires specific planning. Carl will need to list the steps to take in order to bring about change in his life. **First, the decision to seek other employment must be made.**

The basic thing here is that Carl has to TAKE ACTION. To sit around and do nothing probably will draw no result. If he chooses to do nothing, then that is his decision.

Let's talk about *out picturing*. This is like envisioning in one's mind. Thinking about something; dreaming about it. It is wanting something to happen in one's life. We see it clearly, perhaps in great detail. A favorite writer is Dr. Jesse Jennings of Houston who wrote, "Our possessions, relationships, physical and emotional well-being are from our thoughts, our active consciousness."

I often meditate as I begin to fall asleep. I will then visualize what I want in my life (using my conscious mind); the ideas fall effortlessly into the subconscious.

About planning. Whatever you are thinking about is literally like planning a future event. So, I try not to worry so much. When I am looking ahead in appreciation, I am planning. To me, planning is like blessing the day.

Today, I bless the day in all ways. I think good, positive thoughts, despite the external things that may appear.

The external is a vast combination of both positive and negative acts and vibrations that are derived from various places, persons, and situations.

Anyone who has lived can decipher the *appearance* of good and bad. We deal with this constantly. When a negative (toxic) person is in your presence, you are inclined to also become negative because of the magnetic influence they may exert on you.

It is only when you demonstrate a strong defense posture and an opposing position that you can remove their negative state from your presence.

If you don't fight the negative, you absorb it like a sponge. Your mood, thoughts, and actions will absorb those vibrations also. Take a hold of the situation; correct it and you will learn to repel hurtful people and their behavior.

The Ever-Changing Adventure

I have mentioned previously that the only thing we can rely on is **change.** Somehow the status quo (the existing state of affairs) does not exist for long. In a life, change happens--- again and again. Our physical body is a housing for our spirit and soul. The sensible thing for us to do is treat this temple with love and respect.

Change can be scary; it may be unexpected. It can seem contrary to what we think we want. But it can be a call to awaken; to listen and learn from each experience. In many cases, especially in a serious or dramatic situation, there is an opportunity to learn just waiting in the wings.

An important lesson. Here is a true story that provided me with insight about being more understanding with people...

My wife and I boarded our flight at Orange County John Wayne Airport. Fifteen hours and seven-thousand miles later, we arrived at Cairo International Airport. A private van took us across the city to our lovely hotel, which was located near the Pyramids of Giza and the Sphinx.

After touring some of the amazing sights – the Egyptian Museum, the Citadel, Old Market, and the Pyramids – we took a horse-drawn cart around the city. Then we made arrangements to fly to Southern Egypt to visit Luxor, the Karnak Temple, and the Valley of the Kings.

The next day, we sat down to a private breakfast at 4 AM and were transported to the airport. We were first in line, waiting to board our Boeing 737. It was a first-come first-served arrangement. The interesting thing was that the last people in line were boarded <u>first.</u> We were the last two people to find seats. The flight attendant motioned us to take available seats. My wife was seated about ten rows back, and I *alone* had nowhere to sit.

The female attendant said, "Stand right up front, I'll find you a seat." After a bit, she came to seat me. She put me in a row of three in the very front of the plane near the cockpit, where the pilots were about to have us take off. I was in the aisle seat, next to a well-dressed, distinguished man.

As soon as we were airborne, the distinguished gentleman lit a cigarette. I said, "Smoking is not allowed on the airplane." He was articulate and said, "Oh, it is. Let's ask the flight attendant." She came over and said, "Yes, Sir, it is alright."

I apologized to the man and we began talking. He explained how the Egyptian government was organized, that the political regions were near the Nile River, and that Anwar Sadat was the President.

When we landed at Luxor, the attendants instructed us to stay in our seats until the government officers left. THE MAN I SAT NEXT TO WAS THE GOVERNOR OF EGYPT! As he left, we shook hands and the governor said, "It was very nice to meet you." From my seat, I could see soldiers with guns to protect the governor as he got into his limousine.

ME AND MY BIG MOUTH! I learned an important lesson that day about having respect for others. Regardless of the situation, I try not to judge a person. That's good advice... you never know who you might meet!

***

As we sum up this chapter, I share some thoughts I have written down in my journal over the years. I learned that when I did foolish or inappropriate things that did not support sensible living, my body rebelled with headaches, or worry, or other negatives. There was a need to listen to my body; it would send messages that were helpful.

Over time, I eventually learned to speak in more positive, uplifting ways. This took effort. It is easier to be judgmental... we are criticizing, fault-finding, and temperamental. Habits become ingrained; they are not so easy to break.

A very big factor here is this: **The body has 50 trillion cells. Each cell of the body responds to peaceful, loving thoughts. And---your body will respond in healthful ways to those thoughts. It welcomes healing and wholeness.**

Now is that too difficult to believe? Perhaps, but over a long life, I became a believer because I saw results. A great help was the use of affirmations – the statements one makes with sincere feeling and <u>faith.</u>

Faith is spiritual endowment. It is not particularly religious, but it assumes the quality of the divine. We will discuss faith again later in this book. Here is an affirmation I learned:

I am energized. I affirm that divine substance enriches and prospers every aspect of my life. All of my life. Power, energy and substance flow from Spirit as the stream of life within me.

Let's discuss <u>energy</u>. Energy is strength that is required to live, to function as a body (and heart), with physical and mental aspects. Energy is the power that runs this body; to awaken, to walk, dress, take breakfast, to work; to do all the things that are needed throughout our day.

And there's more: To set the mind to accomplish things, to establish long- and short-term goals, to organize the work, and to move toward purposes we adopt in our highly individualized life. I now expand this concept to include that which we *do* with our energy… our determination, the formation of our dreams, and the manifestation of all our desires.

Now, this is important. You may not agree with me, because it might be somewhat removed from any religious or philosophical or ideological belief that you have accepted. If you are open, this affirmation is powerful:

We are all a part of the infinite Energy of the Universe. The Universe supplies us with as much or as little as we ask for and believe that we can have.
> ---Dr. Margaret Stortz, Oakland, CA

So, there are two aspects to this Infinite Energy provision: *1)* All the energy that you want and need is yours, and *2)* you must first believe that you can have it.

It is obvious that the basis for these thoughts must be spiritual. They may be physical, but they are spiritual as well. It is said that if you took all of the assets of the earth – land, houses, diamonds, buildings, everything – and divided them between the 8 billion people on the planet, <u>each person's share</u> <u>would be $4,000,000,000! (That's 4 billion dollars).</u>

Most human beings from any background, religious or not, feel that something is guiding them through the life experience; *the flow*. It is based on a profound item: THE MYSTERY OF THE UNIVERSE.

Sometimes people have horrendous experiences or have deep hurts and disappointments in life. When this happens, they ask, "Is there a God?" They may turn to atheism in that moment, if their faith and spiritual belief leaves them.

The deep fears and weariness of battle-fatigued soldiers in World War II were described in a book written in that time. It was entitled, "There Are No Atheists in Foxholes."

Sometimes, there are no answers to our questions; it is beyond human comprehension. One of the greatest minds of the 20th Century, Albert Einstein, believed that God was composed of Nature, Thought, and Universal Intelligence. He was aware of Man's ignorance when he said, "Only two things are infinite… the Universe and human stupidity, and I'm not sure about the former."

If we are composed of the physical, the mental and emotional, and the spiritual, then these are our components. Life is part of the evolution of the spirit.

We aspire to grow in spirit to the totality of our being. We need to find balance in those components. Within the spiritual, there must be trust of those around you, some degree of planning and accomplishment, and personal power. It is wise to keep your heart open. Be kind and loving. Cherish your family and friends, and be exceedingly grateful for the life. Recognize your strength and value every day you breathe.

~

Attending Pepperdine University

After being discharged from the Army, I went over to enquire about attending Pepperdine College. It was a college then, not a university. It was located at 79th and Vermont in Los Angeles.

I entered the office where I met Dr. Hugh Tiner, the college president. He welcomed me and took me to see Dean Pullias. Dr. Pullias looked at my high school transcript and said, "Hmm." I admitted that I had been a rather poor student in high school, and that I was ready to get serious.

"Tell you what… we will give you a chance, you being a veteran. You will be on probation for one year, to prove you can make good grades."

That was an important day. I soon discovered what was to become a deep love for my life: learning, and getting a college education.

Chapter 9

The Nature of Love

N ow we come to a subject that is exceedingly difficult to describe or practice. You can't see it; you can't have enough of it; you'd like to give it, but you'd rather get it.

I am speaking of love. Love's definition is: an intense feeling of deep affection. If there's anything one wants to hear, it's, "I love you." More songs have been written about love than anything else in the world. I remember this song – we sang it (changing the name each time) to the kids at camp.

We love you Johnny, oh yes, we do. We love you Johnny, and we'll be true. When you're not near to us, we're blue. Johnny, we love you!

Love is not natural; it is learned. And usually, one is over thirty years old before love is truly expressed. June Callwood writes that love can be accomplished only by people who have spent the first twenty years of their lives in a harmonious, loving family.

One needs to have trust in others to express love from the heart. Also, we need to have *faith* – a very important ingredient. Faith in the universe, faith in a Divine Being, faith in our loved ones, faith in our next breath, and faith in the future. Ernest Holmes wrote, "Man has the ability to choose what he will do with his life and is unified with a law which automatically produces his choice."

Love is several things: Love is patient, kind, generous, humble, courteous, unselfish, good-tempered, guileless, and sincere. Love reaches high to its heaven, and drops to the level of its desire. Love has many meanings and is unique for every person. Love can make a person feel like they are sitting on top of the world.

When the infant is fed, he delights with mother; he has doubts when hunger pangs appear and he isn't fed immediately. If she is there all the time, his affection grows; he is loving and happy. The teenager looks to stability and fair treatment and begins to observe family members, and learns about love and affection. The young adult who experiences love in a family will provide traits which result in happiness that will last his whole life.

And then there's the passion of young love. She is demure; she sits quietly in his presence. She looks up into his eyes. He gazes into her eyes and realizes how beautiful she is. She knows the power of silence. Now they share their feelings. It is a time for discovering one other and determining whether or not they are compatible. And also, how much they enjoy each other's company. It is an exciting time…

Mature love is replete with kindness and thoughtfulness, with a sense of cooperation. Now if it is a long-term relationship and/or marriage and there are children, there are going to be challenges, because that is standard. But mature people who love deeply and have a passion for each other, and a strong desire to make it work can sustain their love.

Take a look at any couple who has been at it for twenty, thirty, forty years and more. They have happy lines around their eyes; they have *strength, integrity, and determination written on their faces.* Their union shows great accomplishment. Basic to success for this couple is care, responsibility, and respect for each other and their family.

People who have real love in their hearts, and who bear some of the traits listed, usually have love and respect for *others,* and animals too. And most importantly, they love themselves. The quality of self-esteem in a human being is attractive; lack of it can be disastrous.

What is faith and how does it relate to love? Faith is complete trust and confidence in someone. Faith is a belief in God or in the doctrines of a religion; it does not need to be proved. Faith is spiritual in nature, not necessarily scientific. Neither faith nor love can be measured, or viewed in a microscope. Yet their significance in life is unquestionable.

According to the Bible, humans have been here for about 6,000 years. We have begun to be somewhat civilized and are recognizing our dependence on love as a stabilizing factor. It is necessary for the growth of families, and the evolution of industrial, political, and religious formations of society.

Choices

I have the deep belief that we always have choices in our life. I submit that where life is continually changing *and challenging,* we are not hopeless, and not everything is our fault! But we need to pay attention. The following poem has been reprinted countless times since it was originally published about fifty years ago. It is entitled, *Autobiography in Five Short Chapters*, by Portia Nelson.

Ch. 1: I walk down the street. There is a deep hole in the sidewalk. I fall in. I am lost...I am hopeless. It isn't my fault. It takes forever to find a way out.

Ch. 2: I walk down the same street. There is a deep hole in the sidewalk. I pretend I don't see it. I fall in again. I can't believe I am in this same place. But it isn't my fault. It still takes a long time to get out.

Ch. 3: I walk down the same street. There is a deep hole in the sidewalk. I see it there. I still fall in... it's a habit... but my eyes are open. I know where I am. It is my fault. I get out immediately.

Ch. 4: I walk down the same street. There is a deep hole in the sidewalk. I walk around it.

Ch. 5: I walk down another street.

(Nelson had an amazing life as a singer and songwriter)

You Are the Author of Your Life

By three methods we may learn wisdom:
First by reflection, which is noblest;
Second by imitation, which is easiest;
and third by experience, which is the bitterest.
---Confucius---

Did you know that you are an author – the writer of your book? Yes, you definitely are. You are writing this story. It is about YOU. How you act; the conditions in your house; how you get along with your partner and your family.

Your story is filled with some super events, beautiful days of joy, some wins, some losses, and undoubtedly a few events that you wish had never happened. You probably had a few dreams you wanted to come true, right?

Much of your story is uniquely you. Nobody else could do all those things. You have a special ability; you can be proud of yourself. Oh, and you should be especially pleased about the person you chose to be with and the commitment you have made together.

Your story is special. And there are several possible endings to each chapter; you get to choose the most appropriate one for each circumstance. The beauty here is that you can modify or adjust, as you see fit. We call that a rewrite. Remember, you are the author----of your life!

Some people have said that the soul chooses its next life, who it will gravitate to, what kinds of experiences it will have, and the unique conditions that will occur. I am not sure I can believe all that, but that doesn't mean it isn't true. Everyone has their opinion.

Emerson wrote that one's beliefs and dogged determination are factors in manifestation of events. This seems consistent with the idea of *our thoughts* being a gigantic influence in life's events.

Now I hope you agree with me that you are the author of your life. That being said, I hereby introduce the incredibly important component of abundance known as **radiant health.** I ask you, is there anything more important in life than good health? This is a valuable affirmation for health and one I personally use:

My nature as a spiritual human being embraces radiant health. It runs in my family. It is mine to claim. I recognize that my cells perform their job in amazing ways, serving this body in all its needs, every second of every day. My human heritage of perfection runs through my veins, my blood vessels, arteries, capillaries, routes to my heart, lungs, kidneys, liver, pancreas, stomach, and the rest of the 78 organs. I am grateful for this perfect body.

Do I have to be a medical doctor to appreciate the miracle of my body? Of course not.

It is up to each of us to celebrate the life we want. But we must put our imprint on it. The life we have is uniquely ours. Its design is ours and ours alone. Yes, there is a gene pool with parents, grandparents, great grandparents----all contributing. But we are a *thought pool*, writes Dr. Sally Robbins of Asheville, North Carolina. What we think is vitally important to our persona.

Do we have the power to create the kind of life we would like? My answer is this: To a large degree, *yes*.

I imagine that not many people would agree. And I respect their opinion, whatever it is. But I honor the mind---- the body's engine. The conscious mind decides hundreds and hundreds of details <u>every day.</u> Your conscious mind belongs to *you*---- and my conscious mind belongs to *me*. Individual property.

The basis of my discussion here, and for that matter, my whole belief system is this: good health is our most valuable possession. A healthy body is our sweetest blessing, and our deepest hope is to have this joyful blessing for all the days we live.

The difficulty here is that for most of us, there are days we are sick or are lacking in our performance, or have a slight pain and we fear the worst. However, there are human beings who believe that we are capable of healing ourselves.

This opinion is not widespread, but there have been movements and religious groups that do practice healing. I have great respect for a person who takes the responsibility of caring for their body and recognizing that we have the power within to maintain strength of mind, body, and spirit.

It seems simple enough. Let's take the case of an individual whose lifestyle involves excellent diet and nutrition, exercise, rest, and good habits. The attitude of such a person is mainly positive, his manner considerate and fair-minded. He has a sense of satisfaction about life, mentally and emotionally.

But in reality, most people suffer physical problems occasionally. When such an event occurs, it is painful, miserable and depressing. People are very impatient at this time, demanding medical assistance in solving their issues as quickly as possible.

There is a common belief that most physical ills are initiated by stress. Connected to this stress is the feeling that we do not have control of our lives. And that is when fear sets in, affecting the heart and immune system.

One theme of my book is this:

Every thought and feeling that you have
alters the experience of your body's health.

Influence of others. Picture the day for a man we will call John Smith as he makes his way to his busy office. He hurries past the receptionist. Cheerily he says, "Good morning, Betsy." But Betsy woke up on the wrong side of the bed. She looks up and says, "You look tired, John." He shrugs it off.

John is still thinking about Betsy's remark when he passes the desk of his friend, Jerry and says, "Hey Jerry, do I look tired?" And Jerry replies, "You do look a little out of sorts." Now, what has this done to John's good mood?

People can influence our attitude, and that impacts health. Poor Mr. Smith drags himself through the day and goes home sick, even though he was the picture of health before people at the office talked him out of it.

Mind and body work together. They form a sense of fear, stress, or weakened immune, OR------they create good health and well-being.

Cosmic Religion

This next section is a brief paraphrasing of what Albert Einstein called *Cosmic Religion*. A key factor in Einstein's belief system is one's **needs.** He felt that everything that human beings think or do is motivated by their needs. If one becomes spiritual, they do it on the basis of feelings, (fear, and other emotions).

Mankind moved to religious ideas because of emotional needs. Early on, with primitive people, there was fear of hunger, wild animals, and death. Their imaginings formed a supreme being to which they made sacrifices. Einstein called this *the religion of fear.*

The second type of religious development is based on social feelings. For this, parents long for love and help in caring for their children. This supreme being protects people, and also doles out rewards and punishment. This is the God who loves and provides for the race of mankind. It is called *the religion of morality.*

Scripture tells the story of religious development in the Jewish writings, from the fear religion to the moral religion, then it is carried further in the New Testament. The religions of all civilized peoples, especially those in the East, are principally moral religions.

Einstein indicates that the moral element predominates in the higher civilized groups, but historically, there is always the character of an anthropomorphic god. This factor indicates a limited point of view philosophically.

Now for the third type of religion. Einstein called it *the cosmic religion.* It is in noble communities and gifted minds and is difficult to explain. This concept does not involve an anthropomorphic idea of God. Einstein writes, "The individual feels the vanity of human desires and aims, and the nobility and marvelous order which are revealed in nature and in the world of thought." Cosmic religious sense has three aspects: *Nature, Thought, and Universal Intelligence.*

Einstein did not accept individual destiny; he felt that a person's existence was very significant to the unity of all. The cosmic element is much stronger in Buddhism. Religious dogma and doctrine are not recognized in the cosmic religious sense, and there is no church that is based on the cosmic religious experience.

I realize that this discussion is woefully inadequate to the profound belief system described here. Many of us were trained in the concept of God as an old man in the sky with a beard; He was a person with gender... a *man.* He was kind but would punish if necessary. I was age 3 when I learned about God. I am sure that I would plead to God in some situations, and talk to Him in others; always with deep respect.

When we consider these three components – *Nature, Thought,* and *Universal Intelligence* – they are described in this way:

Nature: the universal power, chaos and order, which sets in motion all the happenings from the beginning to now… each event, large and small, with reason and integrity, despite humankind's lack of comprehension.

Thought: The essence of thinking, intuition, motivation, planning, both conscious and subconscious thoughts, along with vibration, which provide identification and expand communication.

Universal Intelligence: Eternal components of the universe, without limit, spiritually-endowed, set with mass of astronomical bodies, stars, and gravitational pull. For millennia, scientists wonder, study, and learn about the heavens and space.

A significant aspect of the universe is order. Scientists indicate that the universe started out in a highly ordered state. Disorder increased with time. Interestingly, disorder or chaos is part of the order of the universe. Patterns of order appear out of chaos; thus, it seems that chaos is *necessary*. The German philosopher, Nietzsche (1844 – 1900), wrote that chaos is necessary to achieve order.

The principle of gravity is vital, and causes stars, galaxies, and planets to form and hold in pattern. Our sun enables us to have order because the sun forms nuclear fusion. The warmth we get from the sun's rays gives us life. This data provides more examples, which I believe are a part of Universal Intelligence.

Is Universal Intelligence *God?* No one knows. Books provide much information on the subject. There is no way to prove the existence of God, or describe God's characteristics. Nor is there a way to prove Universal Intelligence, Einstein's theory.

In the Universal Intelligence sense, the idea of God is not generally described as a personal God, but an *impersonal* God. "Universal Intelligence" is a descriptive term based on a mathematical formula. It is co-intelligent organization, functioning in an orderly fashion and evolving into more complex forms. They are compatible and reside within or beyond nature. Its wisdom comes from the "Will of God" but is based on human attributes.

There is a "Universal Intelligence" in all matter, continually giving its properties and actions and thus maintaining its existence.

But just because you can't see something is no sign that it doesn't exist. You can't see the wind, love, pride, gravity, electricity, faith, hunger, joy, or thought, but they exist, just the same.

Belief in the divine does not necessarily require a theological point of view or specific doctrine or religion. Emerson wrote that belief in the Divine "stands in some commanding relation to the health of man and to his highest powers, so as to be the source of intellect." This clearly connects one's healing power to a deep-seated belief in divinity... that is, a sanctity, a sense of spirituality; a Supreme Being. ⁓

Chapter 10

It's A Mystery

SINCE THE BEGINNING of humankind, people have asked questions about the earth, the sky, the mountains: "Who made all this?" "Why are we here?" "Why does it get dark?"

About 10,000 years of civilization have passed and we still don't have all the answers. But then starts the Merry-Go-Round. The Big Thinkers go into action… the scientists and genius types. The inventors and philosophers, writers, ministers, and teachers.

Truthfully, *nobody has all the answers.* Yes, people attempt to answer the questions, in a sensible and sincere way. But mostly, human beings simply cannot bring evidence forward with satisfactory answers. So, we adopt the element of **faith.** Faith is complete trust and confidence in an idea or concept.

Faith can be a strong belief in God or in the doctrines of a religion, based on spiritual understanding.

The history of religion indicates the need for explanations for early mankind. With modern technological advances, man still has similar needs.

Good Health Is the Foundation Of A Happy Life

From time to time, life may have trauma and tragedy, adversity, family or relationship problems, or other sources of stress. The road to happiness is not guaranteed; you have to work at it. This chapter offers some suggestions as to how to recover from situations by bouncing back. You have heard them before; here are some reminders, and they are important.

1) Keep fit and have a lifestyle of good health. Affirm that you are in perfect health. Believe it; <u>make it true for you.</u> Back it up with some regular exercise. If you can't do a lot, do a little, but do it every day. Your mental push – your commitment – is really important. Tell yourself that it is a lifesaver----<u>*because it is!*</u>

   Get plenty of rest. Eat proper foods. Avoid fats and sugar. A plant-based diet is best for health. Eat some raw food – 50% would be great – and 80% of your food should be alkaline.

2) Learn to relax. Use strong decision to train your mind. Meditation is a definite winner. Try it----do it every day. It need not take 20 minutes. If you don't have the time, give it 5 minutes. Avoid stress, especially the kind that relates to feelings of anger or resentment. If something or someone bothers you,

have the courage to talk it out. It is wise to forgive people for their hurtful actions. This takes great courage. In meditation, get calm; allow your mind to become still. Let intuition enter. Be receptive and open to every good thing.

3) Be aware of your thoughts. Your thoughts determine your experiences. Remember that you can *choose* your thoughts. You have the right and the freedom to make this vital decision. By this act, you create your life.

4) Face your fears. This may be extremely difficult. Fear is a significant, powerful force with emotional impact. Do not ignore it; it will only get worse. At the culmination of a particular situation, you will be better off.

5) Take time every day to visualize your dreams. Think clearly about each thing you want in your life. What is your wish? Think about it in detail. Oh, and the following can apply to all of the suggestions here: Use the 21-day habit. Commit to something you want to do---for 21 days. It then begins to be an established habit *forever* (unless you decide to let it go).

6) Develop a sense of humor. This requires that you **not take life so seriously.** Now, I will share with you a guaranteed way to stimulate the immune system: LAUGH BIG AND OFTEN! This gets you on your happiness path. Smile a lot; it's the shortest distance between two people!

7) Develop your intuition. A thought that comes to mind and is usually timed for one's benefit. Sometimes called "a sixth sense." Be open to it; it's

like a hunch that a person might consider to steer them in the right direction.

8) Have an attitude of gratitude. No matter what your circumstances, learn to appreciate where you are, what comforts you have, and who you have in your life. People in many countries yearn for something you take for granted... *fresh drinking water.* Being grateful will enable you to have at least two things: more happiness and greater peace of mind

9) Be a loving and kind person. Put forward this idea. Accept it as a high calling for the <u>*beautiful person that you are.*</u> Your body, mind, and immune system will reap the benefits.

10) Develop self-esteem and self-love, for your well-being. Treat yourself with respect. Your life is a reflection of how you regard yourself. So, forgive yourself quickly for any mistakes you have made.

Dear Reader: Your *Number One Job* in the world is to be a happy, whole Human Being. Try it; you will like it!

Some Healthy Stuff

Here's a section of information for living a long and healthy life. First, I will give you the name of a superb medicine you should take every day. It is called *Laughter.* Laughter releases endorphins. In a study, <u>people who laughed often</u> had 65% lower levels of inflammation than those in the control group.

Here are some fascinating facts about<u> smiling.</u> Psychologists have found that even if you're in a bad mood, you can instantly lift your spirits by putting on a smile. Smiles

make a person more attractive, more sociable and confident...
and people who smile are more likely to get a promotion.

Smiling can really improve one's physical health; your
body will have a stronger immune system just by smiling.
Also, the world will love you if you smile more, because *smiles
are contagious!*

About 70% of all diseases are direct choices we make: the
foods we eat; our daily habits; how long we sleep at night; our
use of alcohol; whether or not we choose to smoke; how much
stress we are in; how often we exercise; how we react to our
job, our neighbors, and financial obligations.

If your choices are not healthy ones, and your family has a
history of diabetes, heart disease, or cancer or other problems,
it is likely you will have similar problems. Protect yourself by
modifying your habits; THINK *AND DO* GOOD HEALTH.

I am indebted to Laura Lewis, Certified Nutritionist, for
her book, *52 Ways to Live a Long and Healthy Life* (the Summit
Group, 1993). She has offered much information on diet and
food recommendations in this exceptional text.

A highly touted food is the sweet potato, which is loaded
with beta carotene. These foods containing **Vitamin A** keep
your skin healthy, help eyesight, and promote tissue and bone
growth. Other foods in this category include cantaloupe,
mango, grapefruit, apricots, squash, kale, carrots, and broccoli.
(Cooked is better than raw for most of the vegetables.)

Here is some valuable information about *relaxation.* There
are two types of people: those who are the epitome of calm,
and those who get anxious if they see a cloud in an otherwise
clear sky. In the beginning when humans faced danger, there
were feelings of anxiety and tension; adrenalin flowed as a
result of *fight or flight.* The person ran to escape harm. With
modern society, it is very different; there aren't usually any
clear solutions, and the emotions are kept inside.

Today, stress runs rampant in people. Stress weakens the immune system. Elevated blood pressure can cause problems. People sometimes turn to alcohol or drugs to release deep anxieties. Doctors highly recommend relaxation techniques as a viable solution. The following seven steps used <u>regularly</u> can make a real difference.

1) *Create a quiet environment to meditate twice a day, 15 minutes per session.*

2) *Sit quietly with your legs together and feet flat on the floor.*

3) *Relax every muscle group, beginning with the toes and moving up through your body.*

4) *Keep your mouth closed as you breathe in through your nose. Exhale through your mouth, relaxing with every movement.*

5) *Relax for 10 to 20 minutes, and when you have completed your session, sit quietly and get comfortable; then get up.*

6) *During the entire process it is important not to get uptight if other thoughts are drifting in and out. Eventually, you can train yourself to relax, completely focusing on an object or feelings.*

7) *Make sure you set aside the time to do this meditation daily.*

---From *The Relaxation Response, by Herbert Brown, M.D.*
<u>Exercise</u>. Everybody knows the value of exercise. So, what is this about? It is to remind you… that people who exercise are better able to handle stress.

Endorphins. From a group of "feel good" chemicals of the brain, endorphins are stored in the pituitary gland. They decrease pain and give us feelings of euphoria, and appetite. They also increase immunity. Endorphins relieve negative effects of stress and promote an overall sense of well-being and self-esteem.

Here are some ideas for increasing endorphins: Take an exercise class; seek out ways to give and receive laughter; eat chocolate; eat something spicy; listen to music.

It doesn't matter what specific activity you do as long as you are exercising regularly. You can ride a bike, walk, run, stretch, do yoga, swim, or play tennis. Try to do something aerobic. But do it!

The Power of the Mind

Few people have an awareness of their power as human beings. When one decides to do something and has a somewhat unsure or uncertain attitude, they probably will not see results. But when one has firm intent, with a clear, decisive plan for a specific objective, they probably will have a satisfactory outcome.

People are familiar with stories of patients who've been told they have a terminal illness. They exhibit strong beliefs, **never giving up** on recovery. And they do in fact recover. This indicates the power of the mind. There is no question about illness of the body; it starts in the mind. Nothing manifests in the body except when it is first in the mind. Somehow, among the thousands of thoughts, there it is.

As one changes their mind, they saturate the psyche with affirmatives to offset or remove the negative. Does the scientist accept this technique? I believe that increasingly, the mental is effective. Someone once said, "My thought pool is more important than my gene pool."

Sometimes people who approach old age begin to develop a grumpy personality or bad attitude. Their health is generally worse than other (younger) people. We need to remember that we truly are in control of our health and well-being. Keep a positive, upbeat attitude and maintain connection with those who have similar concerns about health. They can be supportive and help you work through it.

Humans come in two types: the positive person and the negative person. Positive individuals tend to see the best in others or situations, while negative types tend to gripe and complain and then expect you to agree with them. Remember what you give out, you get right back.

We can recall that the conscious mind is the entity----the mental function of deciding things in our life. The subconscious mind remembers all that has ever happened to us, including everything we have ever thought, dreamed, read about, or observed. The subconscious has different names, such as soul, law or principle. Dr. Jesse Jennings of Houston wrote that thoughts require emotion in order to take shape, and that the subconscious is the place that lists and creates the emotions. That is where emotions are added to thoughts.

Life is a series of problems that we must solve, if we can. Your mind is constantly choosing a path to offset or mitigate a problem. The mind applies <u>force</u> when necessary, based on the intensity of the present need. The point is, you have great power, all based on your *passion*.

Focus on one aspect of your life… and be energized by the strength of your powerful mind. You look at a problem, or the person involved, and you act on it after giving it fair consideration.

For many, many years, there has been in use a mental technique that is recognized as effective in manifesting good health, wealth, and other forms of abundance. It is when an individual declares, "I am_____." It is preceded by belief and description, such as, "I am in perfect health today and every day." But, BELIEVE IT FROM THE BOTTOM OF YOUR HEART.

Some people recognize the power within themselves. They state affirmations frequently to remind their heart and brain of this position, and to reinforce their beliefs. Conditioning may allow one to forget or to ignore a belief, even though it is important. It may be called "mental atrophy" and needs constant reinforcement.

How important are thoughts? Does it make any difference what a person thinks? How does what a person thinks affect his life?

One person talks about how life is unfair, people are deplorable, his job causes misery, his partner is an awful mess, and his children misbehave. The other person seems to love life and feels that people are mostly wonderful; has a great deal of faith in the people he works with, loves his family, and is happy and well-adjusted. Now, which one of these persons do you wish to be?

To what degree do thoughts influence life? *Thoughts dictate what is to take place in our lives.* Our thoughts have powerful attraction, and influence our lives in many ways. Every constructive word directly affects our lives. Our consciousness embraces ideas and images; if a person desires health and wellbeing, he needs to express and exemplify good health. He has to believe it with all his heart.

Physicians clearly indicate that emotional stresses, particularly anger, cause physical ills *and worse*. Worry, fear, anxiety, resentment, jealousy, and other emotions are recognized as the hidden cause of our physical suffering. The real cause of sickness is the presence of these negative emotions, along with the frustrations and demands of life. Contributing to this is a fear consciousness, built up by influences from parents and relatives who suffered illness or other conditions.

All the thoughts and emotions we have experienced mold the body in good health-----or create sickness. That is the power of the mind.

Sociologist Aaron Antonovsky (1923 – 1994) searched for the origin of health. He wrote, "We are coming to understand health not as the absence of disease, but rather as the process by which individuals maintain their sense of coherence and ability to function in the face of changes in themselves and their relationships with their environment."

More On Happiness

The great desire people have is to be happy. That starts with good health. A picture of happiness in America would be a contented couple with lovely children playing in their yard, the family dog running around, and all the accoutrements necessary for joyful and pleasant living. Aside from the responsibilities that come with the relationship or family, there are social interests, hobbies, physical activities, and goals. Presumably, the parents are productive and happy in abiding love.

As to love, it is what makes the world go around. Marianne Williamson's bestseller, *A Return to Love*, (HarperCollins 1992), states:

> *Love is the essential existential fact. It is our ultimate reality and our purpose on earth. To be consciously aware of it, to experience love in ourselves and others, is the meaning of life.*

Contentment is vitally important. You are not destined for a happy life unless you learn to be content in all situations. Contentment doesn't result from having everything you desire. It results from showing appreciation for the things you have.

Now we need to add a required factor to this picture: *troubles.* You might prefer to say, *challenges.* I know of no life without challenges. Without challenges there is no growth. Typically, people tend to complain about their troubles.

It could be finances, problems at work, relationship situations, partner difficulties, in-laws, children, or other things that cause us to be unhappy. There are some families who experience problems and challenges that you would probably not want to have.

Happiness comes when we stop complaining about the troubles we have and offer thanks for all the troubles we don't have.

Challenges are here to stay. But mature people will work to overcome them to gain happiness. Happier persons have achieved some level of training or education so that they can function in the workplace, to find interests in life, to obtain a degree of stability and prestige in society. Along with this comes the privilege of leisure time, friendships, travel and other pleasant activities.

Happy people are likely to have some spiritual or religious sense, as well as dispositions to embrace friendships and deep feelings for family connections. Such people are usually admired in the community, and their altruism is demonstrated by participating in charity work, non-profit activities, or financial donations. Theirs is an attitude of giving, cooperation, and generosity, which almost always results in some pretty good feelings.

But there are populations which indicate a lack of happiness and contentment, and it seems reasonable that it relates to a weak or unstable structure, financial insecurities, an inability to reach out to a friendly world, or other problems. We did not know much more (until recently), as psychological studies have been few.

I say again that mostly, our behaviors are a matter of habit. If one is grouchy, it is probably because that individual is comfortable in the role; he gets a benefit out of it and will continue with it until some other habit takes its place.

You remember that if you do something for 21 days, it becomes a habit that stays. The beauty here is that you always have the choice to select what you want. Erich Fromm said that happiness is an achievement that you work at. He wrote, "Happiness is not a gift of the gods."

Admiral Richard E. Byrd (1888 – 1957) said, "… the simple, unpretentious things of life are the most important. When a man achieves a fair measure of harmony within himself and his family circle, he achieves peace."

Abraham Maslow (1908 – 1970) described the state of happiness as being when all physical and mental faculties of a person are at their peak.

Leo Tolstoy (1828 – 1910), in his novel, *Anna Karenina,* described the happiness and enchantment of the hero, Levin after his love had promised to marry him.

Johann Wolfgang von Goethe (1749 – 1832) explained that the heart of happiness is understanding the unique strength and beauty in all living things.

My belief is clear: We are born. We get gifts. Some gifts are pretty clothes or toys or money. Other gifts are hurts or attacks, disappointments, or broken hearts. <u>Yes, these are also gifts!</u> We can withdraw, escape, or work it out. But as long as we draw breath, we choose the course. No one---- but *no one*--- is going to save us but ourselves. <u>*We*</u> have to do that. ~

The Blind Date

My dad was playing ping pong with a teenager and her brothers in Murrieta. Dad said, "You have to call her." So a few days later, I met this young lady on the telephone. She lived with her parents and brothers in Phoenix; I lived in L.A. I asked a few questions such as, "What color is your hair?" (she answered "yellow"); and "What color are your eyes? (she answered "yellow"); and then, "How tall are you? (she answered "yellow").

I knew this was going to be a challenge. Yet there was something in her delightful spirit that was intriguing.

The next week, I drove to Phoenix with my best friend, Mitch. We were to have a double date. We had a few days of fun, laughs, dancing, shuffle board, swimming, and good food. My date was a brunette, 5 feet two, attractive, intelligent, with a wonderful personality.

Three weeks later, we were married. We were blessed with two children, David and Denise. Our marriage lasted thirty-four years.~

Chapter 11

Words, Thoughts, Actions-----They Matter

T HIS CHAPTER CONTAINS some of the most substantial ideas that I have placed in my journal over time. They may be old but haven't lost their significance for reaching the time-honored truths of life and good health.

Bad Stuff: Anxiety and Fear

Among all of these emotions----fear, hate, jealousy, envy, resentment, and guilt----<u>anxiety</u> is the most destructive. It affects behavior tremendously. People who are very anxious sometimes don't even know what is bothering them. In the past, aberrant behavior was called, *fear*. Then as modern living replaced running from a hungry tiger, it developed into the term, *anxiety*. Fear is a reaction to a specific threat. Anxiety is seen as an unfocused future fear. It is a real danger versus an imagined threat

Of course, fear and anxiety are interrelated. The basis of fear is *threat*; the basis of anxiety is *thought*.

Most of the time, anxiety is caused by the presence of change, or the anticipation of change. It is anxiety-causing when people move from their home and what's familiar to them.

One measure of intelligence is the ability of an individual to change, and still remain free of anxiety.

Human beings almost always resist change. When change occurs, man and animal have a strong sense of being vulnerable. The vast changes that took place in the last hundred years – World War I, the Great Depression, the Spanish Flu (1918), World War II, the Korean War, the Vietnam War, and many other horrific world events – have all taken their toll.

As humans face challenges, some are calm and serene, while others are easily disturbed and pained. Individuals are incredibly different. Behind every neurosis is anxiety; serenity in a person probably meant a calm, supportive, loving home. The deep feelings of happiness indicate a background of caring, while mental illness is born out of an environment of upheaval, uncertainty, and abuse.

Psychoanalyst, Dr. Horney, wrote that children are free from anxiety who live in a relaxed home, where they are accepted and adored and when needed, disciplined properly. If children are over-punished, or are not liked or admired, they experience the highest amount of anxiety. Also, if members of the family have unpleasant relationships, it means an increased load of anxiety.

"All negativity derives from fear," wrote author Marianne Williamson, (from her book, *A Return To Love*). We can look at someone who is angry or rude and know that they are afraid, anxious, or fearful.

Anger that is blocked or kept inside can cause tension, hostility, feelings of panic, excessive worry, dread, and other personality difficulties. Children are affected when parents are constantly worried about their financial problems.

Judson Brown, Ph.D. from Iowa State University wrote, "A young child who is punished repeatedly for getting his clothes dirty will likely become an uncomfortable adult when it comes to hiking or other outdoor activities."

Clearly then, we see that experiences, words, and attitudes of family members have a lasting impact on the young.

The development of "self-strength" in people – the innate ability or learned skill of confidence – enables individuals to function comfortably and confidently in life, despite background negativity. This trait of <u>self-strength</u> is directly related to self-image.

Some Thoughts From Allport, Freud, and Maslow

We know that the early environment of a person is very important in their feelings, beliefs, and behaviors... and it influences the rest of their lives. But increasingly, psychologists like Gordon W. Allport (1897 – 1967), Harvard Professor of Psychology, claim that people have the capacity to overcome the less desirable traits of their personality *if* they have the motivation. Individuals have to *want to change* and work diligently at it. They have the ability to make changes as long as they live.

Sigmund Freud (1856 – 1939), a psychoanalyst, believed that lifelong character is determined before the age of three, and that while some changes could occur in personality, no *significant change* was possible after that. This concept has changed now, and the idea of human beings being able to modify behavior is highly accepted and is a part of contemporary psychology.

An eminent psychologist and former professor at Brandeis University, Abraham Maslow, (1908 – 1970) wrote that the efforts individuals make to correct their behavior and grow emotionally, cannot readily be explained.

Maslow is well-known for his theory of <u>self-actualization</u>, or humanistic psychology. This indicates that people can become all that they are capable of... that they are born with the desire to achieve their maximum potential. The study of self-actualization is about emotionally healthy people who reach their peak performance; it is about finding strengths, not deficiencies.

<u>Maslow's Hierarchy of Needs</u>. This study concluded that during their thirties, many people find vitality, and they discover a direction in their lives, which brings a rewarding feeling for the first time. The Hierarchy maintains that a person needs to go through one stage before they go on to the next. There are six steps:

1) Basic Needs---food, shelter, sleep

2) Safety Needs—security, stability, order

3) Social Needs---love, belonging, friendship

4) Esteem Needs---acceptance by others, sense of achievement, independence

5) Cognitive Needs---intellectual fulfillment, knowledge

6) Aesthetic Needs---harmony, balance, beauty

Self-actualization is designed for people to reach their potential and to enjoy greater happiness in their lives. Self-actualized individuals are joyful, highly motivated, energized, giving, and fulfilled.

The self-actualized person has achieved a sense of his own worth; his honesty with himself reveals his integrity. He recognizes and meets his responsibilities, has empathy for others, and is caring toward animals. This human is aware of life, is a kind individual, and has a sense of purpose for living. In fact, he seems to know the *art of living*.

The Power of Gratitude

There is a way to bring more into one's life and it is through *gratitude*. It means thanks and appreciation. The reaction is when we are pleased by what someone did. Gratitude is also setting your intention. When one declares, "I intend that all I do and experience at work with each individual will be peaceful and productive," or they say, "I am appreciative for my job and will be joyful," this gives her *control* over how the day may go. Otherwise, the day will have control over *her.*

Most people would like to have more money (or a better house, or car, etc.). A 19th Century writer, Wallace Wattles (1860 – 1911), wrote *The Science of Getting Rich*. He said, "Many people who order their lives rightly in all other ways are kept in poverty by their lack of gratitude."

Gratitude is usually attached to one's dreams and ambitions. Early on in my life, I was a beginning teacher with a young family, along with a mortgage, car payment, and other obligations. In short, there was not enough money, particularly because my wife and I agreed that she be a homemaker. We both preferred this arrangement.

Our dream was that I become an administrator (school principal). When this was accomplished, we realized how important gratitude is in life; we expressed our gratitude for our blessings every day.

Gratitude is an integral part of the health and wholeness of a human being. Try this affirmation... and state it with deep belief and genuine passion and feeling:

I have been given a great gift----the gift of my physical body. Within my body is my spirit and my soul. I demonstrate gratitude for this gift by treating my body with love and respect.

I listen to the wisdom of my body and respond to any messages I hear. I make wise choices. I think and speak in positive and intelligent ways. I envision myself healthy and whole. Each cell of my body receives loving and peaceful thoughts. With gratitude, I welcome and accept healing and wholeness.

<u>Man on a mission</u>. This is a story about Jack. When he was a teenaged kid, Jack attended a lecture about living right and being healthy. The lecture was named, "You Can Be Reborn." As a young person, he was a sugarholic and had serious health problems, so this speaking event was a blessing.

Jack was so impressed with the speaker that he decided to become a lecturer and physical health instructor. He began to learn all about good health and worked out regularly. He wrote eleven books, including *Live Young Forever* (Robert Kennedy Publishing, Ontario, Canada, 2009).

Jack LaLanne was a man on a mission, becoming a fitness guru and a motivational speaker. His amazing story is one of determination and personal commitment. He was the "Godfather of fitness" and had his own television show for 34 years.

Jack LaLanne had incredible energy and endurance. At age 70, he swam in the ocean near Long Beach, **pulling 70 boats with his teeth** for a mile and a half while shackled. About donuts, he said, "the only thing good about a donut is the hole in the middle."

Jack opened the first health spa and offered exercise and nutrition programs. He called his lectures, "keys to the kingdom." The exercise known as "jumping jack" was named for Jack LaLanne. He would frequently say, "I can't afford to die. It would ruin my image."

Jack lived to be 97 years of age. His wife, Elaine, is in her nineties as this book is being written.

Divine Order

The following quote is from *The Daily Word*, (May 28th, 2020): "Divine order is the glue that holds the universe together. The planets maintain their orbit around the sun. The stars hold their appointed places. The sun rises and sets, and the hours in between reflect this order."

Many things contribute to a person's health and wellbeing. Good health is a basic, natural part of the human being. It is a precious gift; a treasure.

Do you believe it? This is very, very important. Without your passionate belief, it may not happen. The things in your life do not exist unless you believe them. What you want, what you envision, what you think… what you *truly* intend… are in your life, as are <u>you.</u>

An orderly universe is not only sun and planets. It is Universal Intelligence, Nature, (and all it creates); a system of thought for the inhabitants of the Universe. Divine Order encompasses religions and spiritual traditions being present here on Earth and recognizing our responsibility to it.

Jeffon Seely writes, "Divine Order is called the Golden Thread of the universe." The universe is infinite, without limit... there is Essence and Energy, the Spirit that fills everything. Though we do not have the ability to comprehend Spirit, there is evidence everywhere. The Presence enables and creates Life.

There are immutable laws on our earth: gravity, electricity, attraction, magnetism, vibration, and love. Love is known as the great healer.

How one sees and interacts with the universe and views the laws under which we live is very significant. We inherently fear the potential dangers of life so that we are protected, but being aware of the laws of the universe enables us to replace fear with faith. Also, being aware makes life more enjoyable, and one's good health is a part of that joy.

Fear and faith are a single coin; they are opposites. We need both fear---and faith. But do we need to live the entire life in fear? We need to know that everything will be all right. It all works out eventually. <u>This is the atmosphere of Divine Order in the Universe.</u>

Every person senses this atmosphere if he permits himself to. Ernest Holmes wrote, "It would be unnatural for one to doubt either the Presence of God or the certainty of immortality." Further, Holmes said, "there's an interior awareness that everyone possesses. It may have been covered by confusion and fear, but it is always there."

"When one peers out into the stars in the galaxies, when they try to absorb the divine, they will sense something solid and secure at the center of their own being," wrote Holmes.

You can see how one may create her reality through the power of belief.

It seems to me that belief is the engine for the force of life. Enough belief in something makes it a reality. Enough doubt in something makes it nonexistent.

Divine Order is the beautiful and it is the horrible... the growth as well as the decay of life. It is God, Spirit, Source, the Infinite. We can't begin to comprehend the concept of no beginning and no end.

It made minds to think and bodies to exist and Love to bless humanity in all we do.

We Can Change

We can choose what we want to be, and the things we want to do and the way we want to do them. We can be bookish or athletic or adventuresome. And we are always subject to different stages and change.

The only thing we can be certain of in this life is........... <u>change.</u>

Life then, is a work in progress. Let's say a man has a friend who suggests a great opportunity. They are excited and enthusiastic about the proposed idea. But the person thinks about it and says, "Oh, no not me; I'm not intelligent enough to do that. I'm too old (or too scared)."

There's that old enemy, back again. It is FEAR, or his cousin, DOUBT. Go get your dear friends, FAITH and COURAGE. THEY WILL HELP YOU.

Here's a little scientific data: Research indicates that a smile boosts immunity, releases endorphins, and lowers blood pressure. What could it cost you to smile at strangers? Nothing. And it could give you a boost to your immune system. To adopt the habit of smiling will bring a bunch of happy things into one's life… and an increase in **good health**.

To embrace a peaceful way of life is to remove emotions that have their origin in fear and insecurity. In more modern terms, "go with the flow." Another excellent technique is simply to detach from the problem.

"The most successful people have worries, doubts, and anxieties, but they have trained themselves to ignore them," wrote Andrew Newberg, M.D. and Mark Waldman, neuroscientific researcher, Loyola University. People focus on goals that they have set for themselves and continually work on the steps needed to solve problems and remove obstacles. (*Science of Mind Magazine*, March 2019).

A fun fact… here is a little quiz for you: Guess what percentage of our fears and anxieties never happen.

> A. 25%
> B. 38%
> C. 62%
> D. 80%

And the answer is …………….…………….D. 80%

Mark Twain wrote, "I've lived through some terrible things in my life, some of which actually happened."

Emotion is mental energy that is based on feelings. Feelings (like fear, hate, anger, joy, and love) are extremely important. They are deeply connected to our beliefs and our experiences.

Let us say that a 8-year old child sees his father abuse his mother; in heated arguments, the husband hits his wife. The child screams, "Stop hitting Mother!"

That child will remember such incidents his whole life. His deep feelings will likely avoid such behavior; he will never tolerate it in himself nor in anything he observes. He may also attract the behavior... or worse, copy it.

Our best decisions are made in an unemotional manner. Thich Nhat Hanh said, "An emotion comes, stays for a while, and goes away, just like a storm. If you are aware of that, you won't be afraid of your emotions."

In any analysis of human endeavors, we find that there is more to life than the physical. Over time, we embrace the spiritual as well. Yes, we are physical creatures; we are absorbed with and by our bodies. We have a strong appetite for food and water; we want things. We have a strong attraction for other bodies – a mate.

As we mature, we begin to have a more philosophical viewpoint. We start to question life; we need and want answers. We may have had religious affiliations and training----or not. But as we mature, we may draw into ourselves strength, endurance, mental energy, harmony, and a deeper understanding of life. ~

Chapter 12

Two Paths

W E HUMANS ARE not robots. We have been granted the gift of *free will*. We can choose how we are going to respond to a situation.

There are two paths as to how messages come to our attention. One is the path called <u>intuition.</u> Let's define it: The ability to understand something immediately that comes to your mind. You don't know where it comes from; it just appears without notice. It may guide you to go somewhere or do something that will benefit you or someone else. It is a surprise, not a thought-out message. It could be an idea, a solution to a problem that you have, or a warning of some kind.

The other way that messages come to us is through the <u>ego.</u> The ego is there; clever, manipulating, sneaky, negative.

It is designed to punish and instill fear. It wants to make you look foolish and ignorant. The voice of *encouragement* might say, "Don't worry or be fearful – you can do this. You are strong and capable. Have faith!"

Ego would say, "You won't be able to do it. I know you... you just don't have the skills. I warn you, don't try it. You will look ridiculous!"

Which path will you choose to receive your messages and guidance? Intuition or ego? You can decide. You mentally put out the WELCOME MAT. I suggest this:

I hereby welcome intuition to bring messages to me that give me guidance and understanding. I reject and ignore the impact of ego in any part of my life.

As you can see, a major theme of this book is twofold; underline control and self-control. The human being is *star quality*. You can have the life you want, so take control. Be strong, decisive, and determined. Nobody said it was going to be easy. Self-control means choosing carefully; do not be talked into something you really don't want. I repeat: nobody said it was going to be easy.

Perhaps you are old-school; you have been trained in age-old values such as, "Be polite." "Respect your elders." "Obey your parents." "Your teacher (or minister) knows best." Now there's nothing wrong with these standard values, but they should not take priority over your integrity. You are a star!

You Are A Winner

There may have been an absolutely unpleasant event that occurred, but it made you a stronger person. You are wiser for it----and once you admit that, you can begin the pathway of greater wisdom. Your future brightens as you leave the negative behind. (Note: I am assuming there was some negative experience; a painful breakup, bad investment, loss of a job, anything that hurts----just to make my point).

A bumpy past occurred; you will never forget it. Mainly you blame yourself. You never thought you would get through it, but you find that you did! And things look better.

You have discovered strength that you did not know you had. You are a winner!

Memories, Opinions, and Beliefs

Here is a calculation (estimate) of the minimum number of conscious memories of human experiences in a life, at various ages:

Age	Number of Experiences
10	540
20	1660
40	15,500
80	124,800

From life's experiences, we form opinions. We weigh things in our mind and turn some of these into opinions. When strong enough, these opinions become *beliefs*.

A person's beliefs are vitally important. Beliefs define one's lifelong behaviors. Here is a story: A young boy, about 8 years old, is with his mother while she is shopping. He takes something from the shelf and puts it in his pocket. His mother discovers it and reprimands her son, "Put that back! You must never take something without paying for it!"

The boy is nearly in tears. He realizes what he did, and promises not to do it again. The child now understands the concept, accepts the responsibility, and forms a *belief* that should stay with him for his entire life. He has successfully transformed the experience into an acceptable social lesson.

We use a lifetime of experiences to form the way we look at the world and live in it. Our experiences are valuable for our continued learning and growth of wisdom. The real function of learning is to recognize our eternal nature. If we are eternal beings, every experience, every thought, and every event, is important.

This is not a rehearsal; this is the real thing.

Reality is formed for each individual on the basis of belief. We are creatures of great power. If we believe deeply that we have love in our life, then we shall have love in our life.

Ben and Cheri Jamison, authors and speaking duo, write, "Situations in life aren't good or bad; they simply are. Every situation holds the possibility of learning and growth to the degree that we seek it out for its good."

Beginning and Ending

There is no beginning… There is no ending…

We do not understand this. We never will. We can read a thousand books from great minds and we still will not understand it.

About seven thousand years ago, Moses wrote, "In the beginning, God created the heaven and the earth." This first chapter of *Genesis* is a detailed description of the formation of the earth, and indicated that it was done in six days.

Biblical scholars say that this explanation enabled early humankind to understand how life came about. The scholars wrote, "The Spirit of God formed the earth."

Some religious teachings have encouraged the idea of Spirit or God as a person, with human traits and features.

This comes from *Genesis, Chapter 1, Verse 26,* "And God said, let us make man in our image, after our likeness…" It is an anthropomorphic use, not a spiritual application.

"People have made their gods in their image," noted Xenophanes, the ancient philosopher. He said, "The Ethiopian gods look like Ethiopians and the Thracian gods look like Thracians."

Of course, Scriptural references and religious interpretations can be valid as we learn what choices help us to develop integrity and evaluate our reality for living with others; to become tolerant of other people and their beliefs and practices.

Humans have understanding about time and space. One may ask, "What was here before God?"

God – *Spirit* – came <u>before</u> the beginning of time. Life is eternal.

The greatest minds the world has brought cannot explain these concepts. Albert Einstein described God using the term "Universal Intelligence, Nature, and Thought."

Human ills and disease emanate from fear of death… mostly of the body. But intelligent minds, religionists, and philosophers can recognize eternal life as a strong belief, designed to continue life, omitting sickness, fear, and worry; handling challenges with a confident, peaceful countenance.

I've drawn out various opinions in this section. It may be worthy of some discussion to continue this interesting topic. It would certainly make good conversation.

Scientific Stuff: When You Wish Upon A Star…

You look up in the sky and you see a star. But when you see that star, you do not see it. You do not see it *as it is now.* You see it as it was a few years ago. Actually, four years ago or more.

If you view a hundred stars, or a thousand or a *million* stars-----<u>not one exists now as you see it.</u> Some stars may not exist at all, even though you see them. The nearest star to our earth is our sun, and the next closest is *Alpha Centauri,* which is four light-years away. This means that the light it gives out takes four years to reach us.

Say you watch a star every night for four years. It burns out next week. You would continue to see that star burn brightly every night. You would not see it burn out until four years from now.

It takes a long time for a star's light to reach our eyes on Earth. Light travels at 186,000 miles per *second.* This kind of data is beyond our comprehension. We need to ask Einstein to explain it to us.

It seems to me that one purpose of science is to gain some recognition of the power and immensity of the Universe... and to sense that we humans are stars in our *own* right.

There is so much that we cannot explain. As an example: 99% of the universe is unknown to us. We live on this very small place called Earth. It would take about one million planets the size of our earth to fill the star known as our SUN, which provides life here.

If we could end all wars here, every person on earth could have enough of everything to live life comfortably for their whole life. ⁓

Crab Fishing in Alaska

It's 1968... The family is headed for Alaska in our classy, brand new Dodge Camper Van, with sofa that converts to a double bed; single bed over the in-cab engine for Denise, and cot-bed for David. (Everywhere we go, people ask to see inside.) The cover to the wardrobe converts to a table for meals. For cooking, there is also a Coleman stove. We even have pumped water and a sink.

The luggage cases are packed, all set for ALASKA. Truly, this is an adventure of a lifetime. We will drive about two thousand miles to Bakersfield, to Sacramento and to Redding, to Grant's Pass, Oregon… to Eugene and Portland… then Tacoma, Washington, to Seattle… to Vancouver, British Columbia, then a ferry to Juneau, to Yukon Territory, and finally to Anchorage, Alaska.

This day we are going crab fishing; we are filled with anticipation. I rent a wide basket trap, about 30 inches in diameter, tied to a rope. Bait is placed on top. We lower it down gently from the wharf into the water and we wait patiently.

The family goes to the restroom while I fish. Somehow when I tug on the basket, it appears stuck. It *is* stuck! There goes my crab and there goes my bait and my deposit. I cannot allow this to happen. I am supposed to be the leader of this expedition.

I discover a ladder that goes to the water, about 25 feet down. Now the family comes back. Not seeing me, they say, "Where's Dad? Where did he go? DID HE FALL IN?"

I come up the ladder, with basket, rope, and four *live Alaskan crabs*. We head for our camper to cook crab for lunch. Ah, life is good!

Chapter 13

Meditation:
Charging the Battery

WITH BUSY LIVES and full schedules, there is an easy way to reduce stress in the body, lower blood pressure, and calm the emotions.

Meditation is becoming very popular. It is not complicated, but should be done on a regular schedule to be effective. Once or twice daily is good, and you only need 10 or 15 minutes per time.

Find a quiet place; sit straight, and relax. Now fix your stare or look *within*, and close eyes if you like. You are trying to leave all outward thoughts behind – just focus on the silence or recite a phrase.

Breathe slowly and deeply. This is very good for the body. If you are thinking of all the things you need to do, you are not doing it right. What does deep breathing do? It provides extra oxygen to your system, increases energy, and purifies the blood. If you can combine your focus, breathing, and reciting, you will have a strong, valuable meditation session. Repeating some word or phrase is a good addition... such as, "I am strong," or "I am in God's world of love," or "I bless myself and each person in my family," or "The love of God enfolds me."

Appreciate your life; bless yourself as a fine, loving person. Bless your loved ones and all others. The more you bless the world, the more the world blesses *you*.

Change Negative Thinking To Positive Thinking

This is a procedure that reprograms the way we think. It is called, *neuroscience coaching*, which changes the paths we use in our brain. So, what is the change? It is transforming negative thoughts into positive thoughts. What is the big deal, you ask? It is not the same-old, same-old. This important concept has been around a long time (from Mark Waldman, Loyola Marymount University, and Andrew Newberg, M.D. on neuroscientific research, Jefferson University Hospital).

The way we think our thoughts is vital to the nature of our lives. One's specific pathway to an idea, question, decision, solution, plan or concern is guided down a positive or negative road. As one becomes more positive in their thinking and actions, their life begins to change. People around you will respond similarly.

We have talked of the factor of *attitude* before. Be constantly aware of the mind. Your mind makes the decisions.

Do not ignore this – your health could be at stake. *Be a winner.* Be a positive, upbeat individual; surround yourself with people who are like you. Don't let others drag you down.

I would like you to track the number of times you talk negatively about yourself (also positively) in a single day. Test this for 3 days. If the ratio is more than one negative time out of ten, I would urge you to look in the mirror and modify the situation.

Ernest Holmes wrote, "The ability to control your experiences and have them result in happiness, prosperity and success lies in your own mind and the way you use it." Many people have this built-in personal power that is utilized constantly in their lives. I believe, that type of power is *spiritual;* that it is the essence of our being.

Fun With Numbers

There are 206 bones in the body, 60,000 miles of blood vessels, 45 miles of nerves, 78 organs (the skin is the largest), 50 trillion cells, 600 muscles, 6 billion muscle fibers, one brain, one heart, and one beautiful mind.

Each of the 50 trillion cells in the human body has an intelligence that has memory function to keep and maintain wellness of the body. If Spirit has seen fit to create a physical universe for a human being, it seems absurd to consider the body unworthy of attention. My belief is that we are here on this Earth, not able to comprehend it all, yet as Spirit's creatures, we make a determination to live our moments in the best way we can, with deep feeling, integrity, and authenticity.

And we endeavor to gain understanding about the mysteries of life.

Ways To Live A Long And Healthy Life

No one else can take better care of your health and well-being than you can. Charles F. Kettering wrote, "We should all be concerned about the future, because we will have to spend the rest of our lives there."

Walking is the *number one* exercise in the United States. What can happen if this is done on a regular basis? There could be a decrease in blood pressure; a lowering of the heart rate (at rest); lower risk of stroke or heart attack; reduced body fat; increase in metabolism; strengthening of bones; increased energy.

When one has not exercised much and decides to take up exercising, they should do it gradually... and depending on their age, they should consider a doctor's evaluation as to what exercises are appropriate. Most recommendations say 20-30 minutes a day, 3 days a week, to maintain good health.

About one in five people in the United States has high blood pressure. As to the over sixty-five population, more than 50% have hypertension (high blood pressure). It is normal for blood pressure to increase occasionally, but if it does too frequently, it can be risky. There are many things that can be done to keep blood pressure at a normal range...

Reduce salt intake
Avoid drinking too much coffee
Don't have emotional outbursts
Avoid large weight increase
Slow down breathing and heart rate by meditating
Eat potassium-rich foods
(citrus fruit, cantaloupe, potatoes, bananas)
Avoid stressful situations

Use a treadmill and weights
Eat fish, broccoli, strawberries, whole grains
Eat foods with vitamin C, fruits and vegetables

Eighty to ninety percent of all doctor visits are related to *stress*. Some people can let things slide, while others become tense. Can this be controlled? Yes, because most behaviors people have are simply habits.

Early humans – primitives – were faced with life-threatening situations; they learned to flee or to fight. There were tremendous feelings of anxiety, tension, and stress, which enabled man to survive. In today's society, feelings frequently are kept inside and people don't relax enough. There are so many responsibilities: earning a living, paying the bills, (cars, houses, electronics, etc.), driving in traffic, caring for children, attending sports events, church, and other activities.

People who are believers in self-preservation----that should be all of us----would do well to relax in order to improve the quality of life in a modern society. Dr. Herbert Brown, M.D., recommends relaxing twice a day. He suggests brief sessions of 10 – 20 minutes, with these requirements: *1) quiet environment; 2) focus on one thing or feeling; 3) have a positive attitude; 4) have a comfortable position to relax in.*

Eating sensibly is a must for a health-conscious person. One should eat less animal protein and more vegetarian protein. Try to avoid cholesterol/fats. Eat fruits, vegetables, and other produce. Drink plenty of water, eat whole grains, and high fiber cereals. Actually, there are innumerable dietary sources for excellent health. One's doctor or medical practitioner should be consulted as well.

Now we talk about an enemy we love: sugar. There is dependable research saying it is not good for us. Well, we should not consume more than 10% of our daily calories from sugar. Sugar items can make one feel calm, yet eat a lot of sugar and one gets "high." Teachers report that after Halloween, kids get a little wild. Too much sugar and one may have mood swings.

The bad news: Much sugar in one's diet may cause tooth decay, diabetes, arthritis, obesity, and other serious conditions. Remove excessive amounts of sugar from the diet and bring in apples, strawberries, raspberries, and other high fiber items. GO FOR GOOD HEALTH.

I will conclude this chapter by listing four intelligent ideas from an author I highly respect, Florence Scovel Shinn. These are from her classic bestselling book, *The Game of Life and How to Play It:*

> Every disease is caused by a mind not at ease.
> So long as a man resists a situation,
> he will have it with him.
> All disease, all unhappiness,
> comes from the violation of the law of love.
> Hate, resentment and criticism
> return as sickness and sorrow.

A Scientific Look At Happiness

When we search for happiness, we don't seem to consider much in the way of scientific data. The following section relates to information that is science-based, and fascinating at times. Science and research apply a validity when compared to ideas which are opinion-based.

The following are brief statements and descriptions relating to how happiness affects body-health and influences one's behaviors. Most of the data is from a text by Stefan

Klein, Ph.D., who wrote the international bestseller entitled, *The Science of Happiness* (Avalon Publishing 2006). Dr. Klein is a leading science journalist. The book has an extensive bibliography, with over three-hundred references. It was published in twenty-five languages...

1) Joy brings us into a state of perfection while pain introduces us to a low state. Joy affects the body and the mind. Unhappiness destroys the body; happiness strengthens it. Persistent moods of fear endanger one's health because they cause stress. Positive feelings stimulate the immune system.

2) Two neurotransmitters (serotonin and dopamine) are very important in creating positive feelings. But first, let's define. Neurotransmitters are chemical messengers; they send messages to our muscle or gland cells from the nervous system and control bodily functions such as sleep, appetite, and mood... brain activity, motor skills, and others. Communication within the body occurs between synapses, which release the neurotransmitters.

3) A wise person always makes the best of his talents and the opportunities available to him. Dr. Klein states that this is one secret to happiness. (I absolutely agree.) Furthermore, happiness is not automatic. It needs to be worked at as if it affects your life----- because it does!

4) Thoughts and feelings are considered two sides of the same coin. Happy people are more creative; they solve problems quickly. Positive feelings stimulate growth in the nerve connections in the brain. Negative moods are limiting; positive feelings bring us vitality.

Charles Darwin did the first research on facial expressions and years later, his work was continued by psychologist and emotions expert, Paul Ekman. Each found that joy and smiles are innate aspects of humans, not learned. Ekman claimed that feelings and the way we express them are inborn.

Can we make ourselves happy with the aid of our facial muscles? Yes, smiling <u>will</u> make you happy. But we don't feel really euphoric if it's fake; we feel really good when it is a genuine smile. It is hard to trick the brain.

Happiness is not just a coincidence. One has to have good thoughts and actions to achieve good results. This theme is mentioned here, over and over... because if a person is hostile, critical of others, moody (with a black cloud overhead), it begs the question, "What reaction did you expect of others?"

It seems basic, to determine what one wants in their life. Relative to a visit from a famous person, here is excellent advice: *You better not shout, you better not cry. You better not pout, I'm telling you why. Santa Claus is coming to town!* This is straight talk; absolutely true. (Ask any kid). We need to build our intentions every day, brick by brick. The goal might be to <u>become the person</u> <u>you want to be----and truly are.</u>

Perception Is Reality

<u>Perception is reality.</u> Oh? What is perception? Perhaps I should explain. Perception is identifying sensory data. We observe people and events with our eyes. Signals go through our nervous system and we decide what it is. I see a citrus item in the yard; is it an orange or a grapefruit? I slice it and taste it. Now I am sure what it is. My sensory data (what I see, feel, and taste) answered the question and became reality.

We believe what we perceive, and we then accept it as reality. But----it does not always mean that what we see is real.

Dr. Wayne Dyer wrote an excellent book entitled, *You'll See It When You Believe It.* Will we see reality once we perceive it? Which came first?

In the 19th Century, it was believed that one should release their feelings of anger by "letting off steam." The brain was thought to build up pressure, which had to be released. Forty years ago, psychologists found that fits of rage added to anger and increased depression. Neuropsychologist Richard Davidson (University of Wisconsin) said that today we have the ability to control our negative emotions far more than we believed in the past, and those who make this effort improve their health.

One's mood influences mental ability. People's spirits are easily raised by someone in the group who is calm and relaxed. Students who can laugh and are comfortable in class seem to learn more easily. Also, employees who enjoy their work will be more productive.

People who have friends or social connections and family that they spend time with, live better lives. It is important for good health. Lonely people, and those who don't get along with others, do not experience the good feelings that secure people do. Also, having friends actually increases life expectancy. Getting moral support from family or friends is an excellent way to reduce stress.

It has been shown that people without goals or much activity tend to get depressed. Human intelligence encourages us to be active. Stefan Klein writes, "As the body begins to exert itself, the limbs warm up, the muscles relax, and the pulse increases a bit----and it is precisely these responses that reflect the body's sense of well-being."

Everyone knows this: An unhappy relationship affects the health. College roommates who get along well and like each other experience better health and tend to make better grades. Mostly, humans are better served to live together a long time with their partner. It may be more challenging than living alone, but hopefully, it is worth it.

"People are about as happy as they make up their minds to be," said President Lincoln. You can compare people; no matter what happens to some, their happiness level is set. Let's say a person is upset in his situation. The situation changes to where he should be relieved; but----he finds something else to be upset about. It works conversely; things go badly for an upbeat person, but-----she stays positive, adjusting to the new situation. People pretty much stay the way that they are. A cheerful individual stays cheerful; a complainer remains a complainer.

Each person has their own style... their own methods in the way they handle life, and if they get too far out of character, they will be unconvincing, ineffective, and disingenuous. When we dream for some desire to add to our life, we set it in motion; it is on its way. We need to add a couple of ingredients to it: _determination and passion._ Then it can have the deep attraction to appear.

Psychologists say that one's lifestyle and personality are basically formed in the first 5-6 years of life. The four personality types are _driver, expressive, amiable, and analytical._ Is a person better at facts or relationships? Is she introverted or extroverted?

One type of personality is no better than another. Each type is different. Drivers are very strong personalities; they are quick to do things or achieve and accomplish goals. Expressives are big talkers and socializers; are good at communicating ideas and issues. Amiable persons are calm, laid back, and desire a peaceful environment; they try not to upset others. They love harmony. <u>Analytical</u> persons are constantly assessing, making lists of things to be done; sometimes they overanalyze.

Whichever type you are, know this. We are designed to live a hundred years. What will you do in that time? Our lives are affected by our many experiences. An enriched environment expands the cognitive development of the brain. You see some parents who take their children everywhere, expose them to many and varied experiences. Mental expansion draws healthy and enduring lifestyles. ~

Chapter 14

Rules and More Rules

H ERE ARE SIX sensible rules that I've accumulated over the years, that you may like to use for this wonderful, yet complex life.

1) Affirm each day that you and <u>only you</u> determine your self-worth. Don't ever judge yourself based upon the opinion of others.

2) Learn to welcome failure. High self-esteem comes from the belief that obstacles are opportunities for growth rather than proof of your inadequacy or incompetence as a person.

3) Stop expecting other people to understand you. You must decide if *you* like your behavior. If not, then change it without expecting anyone else to agree

with you. Your life will only make sense when you don't need other people to confirm that it does.

4) Stay grounded. Things aren't always a measurement of success. People accumulate material items and they always want more. Your self-esteem is a matter of understanding your value as a worthy person.

5) Keep an open mind. There are no ordinary moments. Every experience in this life is a miracle. Be sure to realize that *you yourself are a miracle!*

6) Make a declaration of some aspect of your life that has great significance. Your health, longevity, career goal, marriage, etc. Olivia De Havilland, legendary 2-time Academy Award winner, declared that she would live to be 100 years old. She reached that wonderful goal on July 1, 2016.

Who Is the Teacher?

I can remember my 7th grade teacher – Mrs. Hebard was truly admired by all. She was caring and sensitive. She inspired me so much that fourteen years later, I became a sixth-grade teacher. I spent the next forty years in the field of education as classroom teacher, vice-principal, principal, and resource specialist.

Who is your teacher? I am going to tell you. It is every person you have ever connected with in your life. It is every event that you have experienced. It is the joys, the sweet moments, the beautiful things that have happened, and the pain.

We are stars in the universe. We are humans, and we are also spirit. There is Something, a Creative Intelligence, a Source, God, Power, *Spirit*----beyond any human understanding----

that enables our spirituality to be sustained and practiced. We therefore are both body and spirit. We need both to have life. As Wayne Dyer has said, "We are spiritual beings having a human experience."

People sometimes doubt the presence of a Divine Being. As humans, we are entitled to question; it is a sign of intellect. But, just because we don't understand it is no sign that it doesn't exist.

Human beings cannot comprehend the Divine Source and we never will.

Let's talk about <u>PAIN</u>. What is the purpose of pain? "What?" you say. "Did you say the *purpose of pain?*" I don't blame you for being upset. Yes, I submit that pain in our life has a purpose. **Pain is our information system, whose function is to wake us; to urge us away from what we are doing that is not right.** If one does not listen, we will likely experience the event again.

As spiritual beings, we can meet the challenges and the pains that life brings. **Pain is our teacher.** Painful disappointments and losses occasionally come into our lives. We direct our behaviors to adjust to the various circumstances. We receive signals as to what is best and what needs to be avoided. If one resists every change, they will suffer.

If a person dislikes going to work, they may be in the wrong job. If one's lifestyle engenders physical pain, it is time to do some serious healing. If one keeps insisting on being correct, winning every argument, relationships suffer.

<u>Try to like and respect yourself for the person that you are.</u> People who have self-respect and a strong self-image, have energy. They have enough energy to share smiles with others, and a willingness to be friendly and kind. These persons are on the road to--------------------HAPPINESS---------------------and----------------GOOD HEALTH------

------------------and a tad of----------------------------
WISDOM.

There are no guarantees with this deal, but the odds are much better if you are willing to compromise a bit. In the 1940's, a book was written, which suggested that one could use four words when people argued, to calm down the situation. The words were, "You may be right." This bestselling book, by Dale Carnegie, is entitled, *How to Win Friends and Influence People.* It has sold over 30 million copies.

Relationships: Conflict, Anger, and Solutions

Let's talk about conflict. If you are under the impression that the absence of conflict in a relationship automatically makes it perfect, I humbly but totally disagree. Conflict is a natural part of any relationship.

People differ; their opinions and beliefs differ – usually greatly – based on their backgrounds and experiences. When an argument occurs, each person reacts differently. One might say, "Well, Honey, I see we are not on the same page on this. Let's sit down together and look at the facts as best we can. List the things we agree on; then the things we disagree on. We will figure it out."

The other person may be impatient, raise their voice, and say, "You know, you are always unreasonable; you want it your way and never compromise."

Try to use Carnegie's phrase: "You may be right." Who knows… it may work!

A mature, thoughtful thing to do in an argument is *listen to the other person.* Look right into their eyes and just listen. After they finish, be silent for a moment; think about what they said. Sometimes, when the argument is over, the air is cleared and things are much better.

The best solution of all is KISS AND MAKE UP!

Actually, all of us want the approval of others. The natural impulse is to desire success, to have people around us who like us and like the things we do. From our earliest experiences at day care or grade school, we wanted friends. As adults, we want the same things. A cheerful disposition is a good start. Life can be enjoyable if you put on a happy face. You are likely to find yourself popular beyond your expectations.

Our thoughts have the power to attract or repel. People are repelled by fault-finders. So try not to find fault in <u>yourself,</u> and do not find fault in <u>others</u>. This will create a cheery environment and attract people to you. Attraction has the power of drawing to you the circumstances that will improve your life that may bring joy, and fulfill your desires.

Forgiveness Means Freedom From Pain

This is a story about anger and forgiveness. It is about a person who is deeply angry with their partner. Matter of fact, this could be you. What your partner did was horrible, but we need not describe it here; just to say that anyone would agree that you are totally justified in your anger.

You have thought of leaving the relationship forever.

How do you think your body is reacting to your hate? While it is commonly known that good health is our natural state of being, when conditions are very negative, the body reacts in ways that are painful.

Here is the truth: You are a creature of love. Years ago, when you met her, you both were so attracted to each other, it was nothing short of bliss. After a date, you thought beautiful thoughts. You could hardly wait until you saw each other again.

What you have here are two human beings who were drawn into each other's arms because of deep attraction and love. This angry person that you think you are is someone else for a short period of time. The ego wants to destroy you while you are down. This is not you.

You need to return to who you really are. To free your body and heart from pain, you need to *forgive*. You do it for these reasons:

1) To dispense with pain.

2) To change the mood to joy and happiness.

3) To bring peace into your heart.

4) To show your partner your moral fiber.

5) To release unpleasant feelings.

6) To show that your relationship is loving and powerful.

A partner's support and forgiveness enable us to be loving citizens in a needy world. By forgiving, have you just won a large jackpot in Las Vegas? No, but you have taken a step toward abundance and freedom in your life.

The Decision

We make many decisions every day. Would you like to guess how many decisions an adult makes daily? (Hint: this was discussed earlier) Let's do a multiple choice:

A. 450

B. 6000

C. 10,000

D. 35,000

The answer is......................................D. 35,000.

Research in 2013 at Cornell University indicates about thirty-five thousand remotely conscious decisions are made in a single day.

We make choices about what to eat, what to wear, what to buy, what we believe, where to work, how we vote, who to be with, what we plan to do in the future, how we take care of our home, car, each other, etc. etc.

Beyond major decisions, there are various levels of decisions that need attention; simple and complex decisions, involving strategies, values, and beliefs.

The decision I want to discuss here is one that affects your health. You awake and greet the new day. You stretch a little; you brush teeth; you get some coffee. You begin to make decisions.

You could make a highly intelligent decision: DECIDE TO MAKE IT A HAPPY DAY. Choose to have positive thoughts. Open up your day to wonderful possibilities, to good news, to prosperity, to joyful events… to *success*. Bless all the activities that may happen this day. And all the people that you will come in contact with. Your mind is this incredible engine; put it to work for you.

Promise Yourself

To be so strong that nothing can disturb your peace of mind.
To talk health, happiness, and prosperity to every person you meet.
To make all your friends feel that there is something in them.
To look at the sunny side of everything and make your optimism come true.
To think only of the best, to work only for the best, and to expect only the best.
To be just as enthusiastic about the success of others as you are about your own.

To forget the mistakes of the past and press on to the greater achievements of the future.

To wear a cheerful countenance at all times and give every living creature you meet a smile.

To give so much time to the improvement of yourself that you have no time to criticize others.

To be too large for worry, too noble for anger, too strong for fear, and too happy to permit the presence of trouble.

By Christian D. Larson

Mr. Larson wrote *The Optimist's Creed* in 1912, and it was adopted by Optimist International in 1922. He felt that people could empower themselves by adopting a strong attitude and practicing being positive. My feeling about this Creed is to rename it **Ten Rules Leading to Better Health.**

The process of being positive in your daily life is not complicated, but requires self-control. People have a natural tendency to dispute or be contentious, because we continuously think... all day, and all night. The ideas come like a flood. We don't mean any harm – it's just that we are basically intellectual, arbitrary, and we need to express ourselves.

Here are my rules:

1) Today is a good day, and I will do all I can to enjoy it.

2) I will be polite to others.

3) I will avoid sticking my tongue out at someone I don't like.

4) I will smile at 7 or more people today.

5) I will compliment people, 4 or more times today.

6) I will remind myself that a good attitude brings a healthy atmosphere for everyone I meet.

7) I will be agreeable, 3 or more times today.

8) If anyone is disrespectful to me, I will give them my big smile.

9) If a driver cuts me off, I will smile and wave, with all 5 fingers.

10) I will make health, happiness, and prosperity my theme for today and for every day.

A Super Day At the Super Bowl

We were lucky to find parking a couple of short blocks from the L.A. Coliseum. It was fun watching the Washington Redskins and the Miami Dolphins do battle. The Dolphins were undefeated, winning seventeen games in a row that year. The coaches were George Allen (for the Redskins) and Don Shula (for the Dolphins).

The Dolphins team was ahead, so we left a few minutes early and headed to our car. As we walked down the street, I saw some people standing together, one of whom was Howard Cosell, the famous sports announcer. We reached our car and started to drive away.

There were absolutely no other vehicles on the street. I drove past that same group of people and decided to pull over. They seemed to be looking intently for their driver. I said, "You need a ride, Mr. Cosell?" He looked at my new car, walked over and made an inspection; he looked us over.

"How many can you take?" I told him four. Cosell and his wife, Emily, got in along with another couple. We later learned that Mr. Cosell had a broadcasting commitment and that his limo driver was late. After we were on the freeway,

Mr. Cosell told us that the rear passengers were his wife; also Dinah and Burt. <u>It was Dinah Shore and Burt Reynolds!</u>

Dinah and Burt were appreciative, kind and grateful. They sent us signed photos that said, "Thanks for rescuing us."

Chapter 15

A Course In Miracles

T HE ROAD TO Peace and the Road to Good Health nat-
urally connect with the Road to Wealth... which is, of
course, paved in gold!

In this section, I share some of my favorite passages from
A Course of Miracles. Later, I will describe what *the Course* is,
and how it became commonly known across the world.

From *A Course In Miracles*:

- I am responsible for what I see. I choose the feelings
I experience. I decide the goals I would achieve and
everything that seems to happen to me, I have asked
for and received as I have asked.

- All healing is essentially the release from fear.

- The highest purpose for any relationship is to reveal the self to the self.

- All seeming change is merely the play of life upon itself and all that happens must happen by and through some inner action by itself.

- Ask not to be forgiven for this has already been accomplished; ask rather to learn to forgive.

- The ingredient which makes the difference between order and chaos is <u>intelligence</u>.

- Your task is not to seek for love but merely to seek and find all of the barriers within yourself that you have built against it.

- You define yourself by your behavior, not by what you say.

- If you are poor and someone gives you money, you will not automatically be released from the mindset which is the conditioned consciousness that created your poverty. But if you earn the money yourself in a fashion that increases your self-awareness, the belief that tied you to poverty will be weakened.

- Perception is the first and most important step in turning the raw data of the universe into reality.

- Trials are but lessons that you failed to learn presented once again so where you made a faulty choice before, you can now make a better one and thus escape all pain that what you chose before has brought to you.

This is the story of *A Course in Miracles*. It takes place at Columbia University in New York. Two professors at the College of Physicians and Surgeons had a somewhat strained relationship; both were greatly concerned with their professional status. Their names were Helen Schucman and William Thetford.

The Course is a book of over 1,300 pages containing a self-study curriculum, which offers truths and principles to help one achieve spiritual transformation. The greatest miracle that one can achieve is the act of gaining a full awareness of love, according to *The Course*.

It was written by Dr. Schucman who said that it had been dictated to her by a spirit guide, she believed to be Jesus. Portions of the book were transcribed by William Thetford. It contains an extensive curriculum, and was written in the late 1960's. One continuing theme is that of forgiveness.

The Course defines a miracle as a choice of *oneness in all living things*. This is a message to forgive oneself by forgiving all things; all people. This is the road to peace.

Marianne Williamson is an internationally acclaimed author and lecturer. Six of her books have been New York Times bestsellers, including *A Return to Love,* (based on *ACIM*), *The Age of Miracles,* and *The Gift of Change*. When she was on the Oprah Winfrey Show, she told about *A Course In Miracles* and it subsequently sold millions of copies.

Williamson indicates that she has been a student of *ACIM* for thirty-five years, and describes *The Course* as a "self-study program of psychotherapy based on spiritual themes." (from her 2012 book, *The Law of Divine Compensation.)*

A Course In Miracles says to relinquish fear and replace it with love. And that love is the basis of a spiritual relationship with God.

I feel that prayer is a personal thing. It is anything one wants to say. When I was three years of age, the common practice was to kneel at bedside and say, "Now I lay me down to sleep. I pray the Lord my soul to keep. If I should die before I wake, I pray the Lord my soul to take."

A prayer should be something that one is comfortable with; from your heart. I also believe that thoughts and words are **energy.**

Let's talk about energy. Words are filled with energy. If you listen carefully, you can feel their vibration. Two people are conversing...

First person: "If there is anything that gets me full of disgust and rage, it is when that stupid governor of ours signs some dumb, crappy bill that brings more harm to people, and wastes money. He steals it right out of my pocket."

Second person: "Well, I read the summary last night, and I think he may have been misled somewhat. You may be right, but there are one or two good parts of the bill that I can live with, because that may help the poor. In the long run, it may save money because of the inflation factor, by issuing bonds."

Negative energy words	Positive energy words
rage, disgust, stupid, dumb, crappy, harm, wastes money, steals	good, I can live with, help the poor, save money, you may be right

Generally, each word has intrinsic value attached to it. Example: *antagonistic* sounds argumentative, but *cooperative* sounds like we are going to get along.

Richard and Mary-Alice Jafolla are Unity Church authors. They said that when soothing words are spoken to a frightened child, he calms down. "Soothing words release soothing chemicals in the body." This shows the power of loving thoughts expressed. (from their book, *The Quest*).

In a scene from the movie, *A Farewell to Arms*, with Rock Hudson and Jennifer Jones, a soldier and a priest are playing chess. The soldier asked, "Father, what if you find out there is no God?" The priest replied, "Well, I shall keep the bad news to myself." (Screenplay by Ben Hecht, 1957)

I Believe

Over the years, with thanks to my parents, I have learned to seek knowledge; also, with thanks to the teachers I had in school, and to my Aunt Hilda and Uncle Josh. Pepperdine University and other colleges I have attended helped me grow spiritually. *And I'm still learning!*

Here are seven items of belief that I think help one to experience good health and happiness... to live a good life.

1) The Deity. There is no *man-god* up in the sky. The Deity is beyond human understanding. But there is Source-Energy... Spirit, in everything... and unlimited Intelligence. Each person may choose the terms they use to express their spirituality. Through our discoveries, we experience <u>true freedom</u>. Why? Because we are here to learn and grow, and contribute to the collective human consciousness.

2) Kindness, compassion, openness, and love form a healthy approach to life.

3) Certain principles and spiritual laws enable us to better our life conditions.

4) Strong, determined thinking with a positive attitude, has great value, enabling us to enjoy prosperity in health and abundance.

5) Heaven and hell are states of consciousness, not afterlife destinations.

6) In this life experience, I learn all kinds of valuable lessons, all designed to expand consciousness.

7) Life is eternal; immortal; forever expanding the soul.

Interesting Data: Schools

I came across this information, provided by Robert Reasoner, former super-intendent of Moreland, California School District...

1. What % of children 5 years old (CA) have both parents working?

2. What % have parents with separation, divorce, or remarriage?

3. What % (high school-aged) are not living with two parents?

4. What % are born out of wedlock and have never known a father?

5. What % were born with their mother's effects of drug abuse?

6. What % of high school graduates will have been molested or abused?

7. What % of kids come from families with alcohol or drug problems?

8. What % will contemplate suicide?

9. What % of girls will become pregnant before graduating?

Answers:	#1	68%
	#2	50%
	#3	68%
	#4	24%
	#5	24%
	#6	25%
	#7	25%
	#8	30-50%
	#9	10%

These statistics are dismal. What can be done about this? I care deeply for our youth… we must give them a better chance in the world.

The Wealth Department

Mainly, we have discussed good health and ways to achieve a happy, fulfilling life. One in which people can enjoy their treasure. Also, we want to avoid stress in our life because stress is the enemy of vibrant health and true happiness.

We have not given much attention to the subject of wealth. When one enjoys good health, they are rich. Having good health and vibrant energy are blessings indeed.

Some highly desirable goals of wealth are having lifetime income. This enables one to live without the stress that generally accompanies a struggle to pay bills and earn enough money to cover expenses. The goal of retiring earlier than usual gives opportunity to travel and do things one has wanted to do.

Achieving financial security gives people peace of mind. It allows us the ability to help those less fortunate… to pay for college and other opportunities for children. The accumulation of money and assets make life more enjoyable for people as they make plans for their lives. But money means different things to different people. Also, it may be less or more important at certain times. The following list of references could be helpful as people set and achieve their goals.

I found three excellent texts (all bestsellers) on wealth. Of course, there are innumerable resources available at libraries and book stores, and on-line:

1) *The Road to Wealth*, by Suze Orman, Riverhead Books, New York, 2001 695 pps.

2) *Money, Master the Game*, by Tony Robbins, Simon and Schuster, New York, 2014, 650 pps.

3) *Think and Grow Rich*, by Napoleon Hills, Ralston Society, 1937, 198 pps.

The Seven Laws Of Nature

An article written by Paul Turcotte (*Inside Destiny*, 2011) explains this 5,000-year-old wisdom which says, there's a natural *ebb and flow* to life. It is necessary to accept what life is and to go with this natural flow of energy. These Laws of Nature give us a structure to life. They can be relied on; we feel a sense of confidence. We are not like a leaf in the wind, falling... being tossed about, without any considered thought, plan, or purpose.

Life----and everything in it----has purpose and integrity. We don't just live, then die in oblivion. Our creation – our existence – is significant. The events, the narrative, and the characters, are a puzzle, not to be totally understood, but each piece is important.

For ten-thousand years of recorded history, humankind has attempted to explain the mysteries of creation, the nature of the universe, the science of the earth, and spirituality. An example of an earth mystery is: why does earth have this abundant amount of water when no water exists anywhere else in our solar system? There are some theories, but scientists are still working on this.

Here are the 7 Laws of Nature…

1. The Law of Attraction and Vibration. People attract the energy they have. Each individual has a personal and constant energy. Positive people attract others who are like them, and think and act in a similar fashion. Thought is energy. A thought goes out to someone; it can be magnetic. There could be a meeting of minds.

Every person has vibrations, which are positive or negative. We are able, at any time, to select our thoughts and the qualitative nature of them, which can have emotional impact, depth, or character. They can be serious or humorous. *We are what we think.*

The energy you give off is what you will receive. For the purpose of your own health, you need to omit, to the best of your ability, the negative. Feelings are extremely important; how you feel about something or someone is the basis of the attraction or repulsion.

2. The Law of Polarity. Everything has an exact opposite. There are two sides to everything in the world; a coin, political parties, an engine is on or off, one's health condition, the weather, the placement of something, one's financial position----joy or sorrow, up or down, hot or cold, smile or frown, laugh or cry.

Accept both sides of a situation, and life will be smoother. Also, you may see that there is value in the other side. It is usually very difficult to see both sides. Let's say that your homeowner association raises the monthly dues. You and others object and ask for reasons why the board took this action. The board does not give any reason.

This causes a bitterness in a tense situation, which really needs a solution. This would mean being courteous and open to communicating. There are lessons to be learned and possibly, a solution could be reached in time. Is there value in both sides? Of course.

Try to see the positive in every situation. Acceptance of the information and those offering it, is a great achievement and will be significant to one's health.

3. The Law of Rhythm. Everything is moving in rhythm. When we reject, argue, resist, or change things in an unpeaceful manner, we create obstacles. We would do better if we go with the flow----remain calm----try to accept and see both sides of an issue. This is a sound procedure.

Maintain your goals, dreams, and visions in the business of life and in all areas. Exercise self-control; be confident, not fearful. Alleviate the unpleasant feeling of fear by breathing slowly and deeply. Be in a quiet place. Think pleasant thoughts; envision a peaceful place such as a mountain or lake.

4. The Law of Relativity. Everything is relative. We are always comparing things. Look at something as it is. Like *you.* There is nothing in this world that you are more aware of than *yourself.* Do not compare yourself to the past and do not compare yourself to another person. The work you currently do should not be compared to a different job in the past. Do not be entrapped *by the ego* with such thoughts as, "I'm not good enough" or "I can't do the work they expect of me."

Look at things without judgment, particularly when evaluating yourself or your performance. Get used to the idea that you are enough; you are perfect as you are. Comparisons are never what they seem.

Sigmund Freud described aspects of people's mentality, called the *id, the ego, and the super-ego.* This was his theory of personality. They are not part of the brain, just systems that develop at different stages in life. This theory is a study of its own. I have mentioned it here because it frequently attempts to disrupt and discourage us from our intentions to succeed.

We need to avoid that discouragement when it occurs. We are stronger than those aspects of personality... and need to attack back with positive power and statements such as, "I can do this!" or, "There is no reason that I can't succeed on this project," or "I will make every effort to be the best I can be!" Sometimes we need to remember that *honest effort never goes unrewarded.*

5. *Law of Cause and Effect.* For every cause, there is an effect. For everything you do, there is some kind of reaction. An action brings a reaction. This is basic to the universe. Send out good thoughts to someone and you will get good things in return. Send a hostile or angry thought to someone and you will receive the same kind.

You have power as a human being. Your thought structure is balanced, supported, and enhanced by tremendous brain power. Use your power carefully. All that occurs is perfect. It just doesn't seem perfect, with all the negativity that appears in the world. Even our blessed country, the United States, is beset with large problems in the areas of a pandemic, social and political issues, and divisiveness in the nation in an election year.

Know that all these challenges have purpose. Things are the way they're supposed to be. For the sake of your health... the quality of your life, and peace of mind... begin to accept the circumstances, the people, and the conditions of it. The sooner, the better.

The vicissitudes of life – the ups and downs – are to be expected. They are inevitable. Situations may get better or they may get worse. Your power is within you. It is your choice as to how to proceed in your specific area of activity----your home, city, family, and job.

But-----------NEVER EVER GIVE UP. NEVER.

6. The Law of Gender and Gestation. The components of the universe are male and female; two very different energies, both necessary. Male domination in the past allowed such inequities as viewing women as "property," but social progress developed with time. In today's world, women have surpassed men in many areas. This may be considered a gestation period, showing growth and development.

It takes time for a thought to manifest into a physical element. A young man dreams of the beautiful car he wants. He envisions it; how he will take the wheel, how his friends and girlfriend will admire him and his new car. He is determined to take delivery soon. He is working hard at his job to save as much as he can.

It is entirely natural to have things manifested in your life when the dreams get powered by your strength of will and determination. A gestation period can be applied in situations of high interest – your thoughts and dreams. Add some patience to the equation, and manifestation may be in the near future.

7. The Law of Perpetual Transmutation of Energy. The universe has energy fields that constantly flow. Energy is never created or destroyed; it moves from one form to another. *Transmutation* is the action of changing into another form.

All energy that is in motion will eventually become physical. I believe what this means is that our thinking can manifest reality. This is basic metaphysics. Ernest Holmes wrote that thoughts are things. The Law (of Perpetual

Transmutation) indicates that it does not judge thoughts; if one thinks about something they want in their life but also thinks, "oh, it probably won't happen," one thought will cancel out the other.

Thoughts that are random or are deemed unimportant will be discarded. But if there is consistent focus, there may be an effect. What your mind truly believes will contradict a thought of lesser belief. The thoughts our mind takes hold of are those thoughts that are consistent. When we worry, we think about the things that bother us far more consistently than our wish list, so worry dominates the wishes.

This relates to built-in, long-term habits. If you are a worrier and you spend 90% of your time worrying or having fears, it may be very difficult to get your dream going. I've heard it takes twenty-one days of serious thinking and concentration to change a habit or establish a new belief.

Be sure that you concentrate on the things you truly want to manifest in your life. This is like saying, "Be careful what you wish for; you may get it." You need to think positive thoughts, not negative thoughts.

Now for more straight talk. I've listed some age-old techniques that have been around for many years, to help transform ineffective thinking to manifest your dreams and desires:

> Use positive affirmations
> Use visualization techniques
> Form a vision board (look at it 5 times a day)
> Read inspirational articles and books
> Listen to soothing music
> Act as if you already have what you desire
> Be grateful for the good things in your life

Chapter 16

Affirmations, Philosophy, and Wisdom

I WANT TO begin this chapter with an affirmation: *I am conscious of something that directs me in my life. I call it Infinite Wisdom. Whatever I ought to know, I shall know. Whatever I ought to do, I shall do. Whatever belongs to me will come to me. My every thought and decision is molded by Intelligence and expressed through Law in my experience.*

I need to remember the powers that I possess and can use every day of my life: the power to think, the power to analyze, the power to decide, and the power to evaluate a situation and act in accordance with the choice I make. If I select a life of prosperity, I can have it. I can have a life without prosperity should that be my choice. The Creator has given me *free will.*

I know that freedom and joy are mine. If I declare them, they are mine, with earnest effort and intelligent action.

Change – we did not see it coming. It can be a wake-up call. Change results in better ways of living, despite the sudden and sometimes shocking event. It is often a negative experience. But----wait a period of time, and you will see that it was a blessed improvement, all for the better.

Every change has a beginning and an end. We can choose what we emphasize. Affirm this: I envision the best for myself and for others. I intentionally see beauty in the faces and hearts of those individuals around me. I see the best in people. (This is not always easy.) I honor our differences. We may not agree, yet I can recognize the oneness in human beings.

Cells Transmit Signals. If your cells give the signal that you are vibrant and healthy, you are a fortunate person. The mind receives the signals, then proceeds to implement the order. If thoughts of illness, negative emotions, anger and the like dominate the neurotransmitters, established beliefs will take over and give us what we have asked for. Beliefs about illness are seeded in the first six years of life, when they are downloaded into the child's subconscious.

On Balance

Walt Whitman said, "The gift is to the giver and comes back most to him---it cannot fail." He was saying that the giver of the gift receives the most pleasure. I agree.

The universe is in balance; it gives and receives. Nothing can leave any point without an equal something returning to it.

Do you accept the gifts you have been given? If someone gives you a gift, do you happily accept it? Do you think you deserve it?

Do you love and respect your body, or do you think you are self-centered and narcissistic? Here is a reminder for all of us:

I have been given a great gift----the gift of my physical body. It is the housing for my spirit and soul. I show gratitude for this gift by treating my body with love and respect.

My vision for me is all good things, vibrant health and energy. Each cell of this body is healthy and whole... and at peace.

Every experience we encounter shows us some truth about ourselves. We are here to unfurl the truth of what we already are and to discover that God is within us.

Now, I have the realization that we are not all on the same page. And that's okay. One person is deeply religious or spiritual; a second believes there *is* no God; and the third is not sure *what* he believes. Still others in the world revere very different practices from our own. Tevye, from *Fiddler on the Roof,* talked to God many times every day. I say, whatever works!

Some say, "That was an act of God" to describe an uncontrollable event; others believe that God is an internal awareness. Our spirituality is as unique as our 8 billion bodies are different. Our feelings and beliefs are ours and ours alone.

Perhaps the best advice is what Eugene Holden wrote about how to live in this universe (from *Guide For Spiritual Living):* "Today I am a neighbor to all and a stranger to none. The universe holds us all in loving embrace."

<u>Ageless Being.</u> The philosophy we will discuss here may be far different from yours, but I want to discuss it. I do not

hold the belief that we live this brief moment, a hundred years, then die and go away forever. Did Universal Intelligence (Source, Infinite Presence, Spirit, The Deity, Supreme Power, The Divine, God, Creator) set such a brief experience as the life?

You are an ageless being. You are timeless. Your unique soul is an individualized expression of an eternal life. For an expanded understanding of the concept of multiple lives, I recommend any books by Hugh Lynn Cayce – son of Edgar Cayce – about his father's readings on reincarnation. (We will discuss Edgar Cayce again in the next section.)

<u>More on Gratitude.</u> Here I go again, writing about gratitude. If one could place gratitude on the top of every list… the first of all the thoughts one has, and ten times every hour, the smiles would appear and a person would realize his or her fortune.

Look your best at every age and be happy and grateful that your body is healthy and vital. WAIT---Alright, you say you are in pain; you have health issues; you can't believe there is a God because horrendous things have happened in your life. There are terrible struggles. Yes, fortunately, that is true. Let me repeat that: Fortunately, that is true. Now you may have some question about my sanity. The truth is that the trials and tribulations of this life are designed to have us grow and mature.

God could have said, "All humans will be born with everything they could ever need or want; they will never experience pain or hurt, or worry about anything. Every need and desire will be met immediately." Apparently, that is not the plan.

You know that things could be worse. The thing to remember is this: **The response for today is the determiner**

for tomorrow. If you moan and complain and have regret, you are destroying the possibility for change. To go with the flow. Take a chance and smile; be grateful and happy, and you are going to see some good coming your way. <u>But you have to believe it with all your heart.</u> At all times in your life, you are your beliefs. *You are what you think.*

Every physical form passing through time will change shape, age, and eventually pass into another dimension. Look in the mirror and be kind to yourself. It is not easy to be here, but this life is not designed to be easy. Affirm this: **I am grateful to be alive!**

Spirit is everlasting. You will continue your work in the spiritual realm after your time is done. The basis of life on earth is <u>change.</u> The universe is always conspiring for our good, so whatever change is taking place is ultimately for our good. There are lessons to be learned… deepening to be done, and inner transformation to take place. This is the role of change.

You Are the Architect Of Your Happiness

As you learn to trust and have faith, the whole process of earthly life improves. So, look for the good… praise it. Try to see the best in yourself and others.

Your thoughts are things that create the conditions of your life. Choose your thoughts wisely, for you are the architect of your happiness. You are probably not totally aware of the power of your will. Spirit has set will power in us; we are able to direct the events of our life, to a great extent.

Edgar Cayce (1877 – 1945) was an author and clairvoyant. He answered questions about healing, nutrition, reincarnation, and the afterlife. He maintained that "all mortal sorrow in human beings come from our misuse of free will, given to us by our Maker." Cayce wrote, "God does not sit in judgment, give punishment, nor give awards to a favored few." He understood that God relinquished such privileges when he gave every soul freedom of action, choice and decision.

Another belief Cayce was definite about was that nothing surpasses the rule of man's own will power. This is opposite from a belief in destiny or fate. Do you believe there is a hidden power that will control what happens to you in the future? Do you believe that your future is pre-ordained... that the course of events of your life are inevitable?

No, we don't have much control when we are two years old. Father or Mother will grab our hand to keep us safe. And at age five, Dad will keep us from falling off our first ride on a bicycle. But as we mature, we yearn for our freedom.

As we go through the years, day by day, we make our discoveries. We attend school and connect with teachers and friends... then graduation... getting advanced training, jobs, promotions, etc. It brings the joy of success----and occasionally a correction or two. We discover love and affection, along with some valued relationships.

Our mind is continuously seeking answers for us: is there a plan for my future? What should my main goal be now? Do I need more training? We don't comprehend our own power, but we sense somehow that we will be successful in solving some nagging problems and finding our way to happiness.

Life's lessons can reveal many things. We have many teachers along the way, not only from a classroom. It could be a friend, a boss, a neighbor or parent, a clerk, or a lover. Look at this individual as a valuable teacher. Sometimes it seems that these "teachers" have, as their sole purpose in life, just one task: to make us miserable. They somehow reach our emotions and *make us crazy*. They can destroy our morale and lead us into anger.

But the truth is they are valuable because these teachers offer some significant lesson, such as forgiveness, patience, understanding, or compassion. So be grateful they are in your life.

Accept the lessons that you are given. There are going to be setbacks. And disappointments, and even heartbreak. But----get on with life. Life provides us with continuous opportunities. Did you fall off your horse? Get right back on; make the correction and go. Remember: Free will is always stronger than pre-ordained destiny. You are never so encumbered with errors of the past that you can't make the necessary comeback.

Who Is Responsible For You?

You and *you alone* are responsible for your life. These are some practical thoughts and ideas that relate to life. Really, they are principles…

We have been given free will. We have the power to determine what we want to do in this life. We choose our attitude about work. We choose the habits for our daily life, the foods we like, the number of hours we sleep, etc. We have innumerable choices.

Human beings are incredibly curious. How did the earth form? What is God? Can we prove His existence? Do we look like God? Why is there so much suffering here?

The problem is, we don't know the answers. Early in our lives, we form opinions through parents and others; we get ideas from teachers and friends, and at church, and through reading, watching television, and going to the movies.

The process may take years, but we and we *alone* decide what beliefs we will have.

We may hear about an idea or philosophy that is appealing to us or captures our interest; we want to know what it is. Perhaps others we know have mentioned it to us, and we want to learn more so that we can intelligently discuss it. This takes us into our next section. It is something currently in the news. **It is here strictly for the purpose of discussion.**

Food For Thought

Socialism vs. Capitalism. Nothing is true unless it works for you, and you have substantial understanding about all aspects of it. Socialism is a system of economics where production is controlled by the government, and funds are distributed to people by the government. Originated by Karl Marx who said that Socialism would be a step followed by "a perfect society, classless and stateless----called communism."

Capitalism is free enterprise, with the central idea of private property... that individuals and corporations have the legal and moral right to own property and accumulate wealth.

My personal experience is that I had a father, grandparents, and uncles who emigrated to America. The opportunity here, in the United States, is magnificent and is available to those who have initiative and ambition, and a willingness to learn and work hard.

Those people in my family were successful and highly respected in their communities. They became U.S. citizens, learned English with excellence, and embraced this country as did millions who came here before them.

The beliefs we adopt are important and require careful study, utilizing thinking and feeling.

The use of NO in important decisions. There is a great deal of power in the word, *no*. Suppose that you have something in your life that you want to get rid of. Eliminate it by stating to the subconscious mind in specific words exactly what you wish to delete. Be sure that you want to remove it from your life. Say it out loud in a clear voice, and feel it strongly. Take several minutes to make it jell. What you state in the subconscious-----mentally and emotionally----must act for you. And do not undo your declaration with doubt by saying, "this probably won't work." Your assuredness and your clarity are important.

Communist Curriculum

As you certainly must know, this world with eight billion people, has eight billion opinions. There are about two-hundred countries, all different. We enjoy a democratic form of government, but here is an example of Communism, a system far different from ours.

Communism is supposed to spread the wealth to help the poor. It has been tried many times. Information is withheld; the people are deceived. No one owns anything and they are told where to work. The Communist State says they will care for the people and tells them they should be loyal to the government.

Communists mislead in order to gain power. Children are especially vulnerable...

A man brings two similar plants into the classroom. They are placed on the window sill where they can get sunlight and air. He says, "This first plant will be taken care of by the State; it will be watered and fed properly. This second plant will be taken care of by God."

Time passes. Three weeks later, the man returns to inspect the two plants to see how they grew and if they bloomed. The first plant is verdant and attractive. The second plant is dead.

The man says, "The State takes care of us the way this plant is cared for; this dead plant shows you that there is no God."

Each of us must decide for ourselves. I cherish our freedoms here. We can share our thoughts, stand up for what we believe in, or do nothing.

One final thought in this discussion: **Nothing has ever happened to you or taken place around you that was not the result of your subconscious mind.** (from *The Power of Decision*, Raymond Charles Barker, 1988)

The Pilot

During art period in school, I always drew a picture of an airplane. Nothing else; just airplanes. When I joined the Civil Air Patrol, I could occasionally go up in a small plane. It was really fun.

When my kids were all grown up, I made the decision to learn to fly an airplane. I came home and said to my wife, "Guess what! I have decided to go to Ground School and learn to fly. Ellie said, "Did you say, fly?" "Yes," I replied. She said, "Let me get this straight…You are going to fly an airplane?" I declared, "That's right."

Orange Coast College offered an excellent ground school class, so I signed up. After completing that course, I attended the Cessna School at John Wayne Airport. Six months went by of intense study and flight lessons.

The big day finally arrived. A Federal Aviation Administration (FAA) flight examiner went up with me, put me through a series of various situations involving speed, altitude, control, and… stalls!

When we landed, the examiner said, "Congratulations, you passed." I flew the Cessna 152 and the Cessna 172 over the next 12 years. I flew to San Diego, Bakersfield, Santa Barbara, Catalina (oh, that was exciting!), and other small airports around Southern California.

I discovered, there's no way a pilot like me can fall asleep while flying an airplane, because most of the time, I was terrified! (in a good way.)

Chapter 17

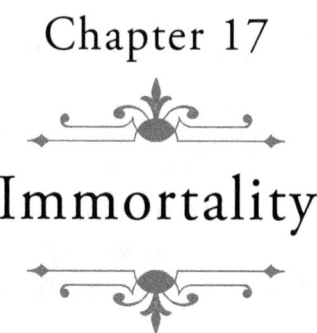

Immortality

IMMORTALITY IS ETERNAL life, existence forever. Certain scientists and philosophers have said that immortality of the human might occur someday, suggesting that it may be achievable in these first few decades of the 21st century.

Many people have theories about an afterlife, reincarnation, and eternal life. There are individuals who say, "Why would you want to live this life again?" There are many examples in Greek mythology of gods who are immortal. And there are those who view the experience of life as precious, despite its challenges.

The literature offers a good deal of information, theories, near death experiences, and other accounts, which describe the idea of an afterlife.

Also, the concept that "there is nothing to fear" appears in religious doctrine, spiritual guidance, psychology and in other writing.

Near Death Experiences

My friend and I have a talk. Mike says, "I believe that there is an afterlife." I reply, "But there is no evidence." He counters, "There is much evidence. There are thousands of *NDE's* (near death experiences), the Cayce writings, books by Albom, Klein, Atwater, Abanes, Fox, Long, Zukav, and numerous testimonials."

Then I say, "But there has been no communication with anyone in the afterlife." Mike replies, "I'm not so sure about that." (we both laugh).

The age-old questions, the claims made by psychics and clairvoyants, the mysterious phenomenon, all provide information to our minds. For centuries man has been seeking answers… is there an afterlife? Is there reincarnation?

Turn the coin over and appears a concept called faith. "Faith is the substance of things hoped for, the evidence of things not seen." (from Hebrews, Chapter 11).

My belief system is activated. Despite the challenges of this life – the occasional disappointments, the loss of loved ones, the tears – I have begun now to learn about the nature of life, the beauty of it, the truth, the gifts; the known and the unknown.

I appreciate these precious days. I want to live additional lives in search of joy and happiness, and to learn more about love and life.

My time here this time is just a blink of an eye----a mere 100 years. I have created a different term. It is *newlife.* Newlife means an individual who has entered a brand-new life, after living a previous life. In effect, a *newlife* is an afterlife.

Perhaps funerals in the future will be celebrations in which we send our loved one blessings as she enters newlife. When I was in the army, I was stationed in South Korea. We saw people at a funeral, dressed in white, solemn and respectful, but not depressingly sad.

Buddhists believe in a cycle of death and rebirth. Through karma, they hope to achieve an end to all suffering.

Death Is Not the End Of Life

Arguable, the most pronounced fear in life is the fear of dying, and the idea of the total end of life, of oblivion forever. My belief is that life is eternal, and a continual adventure. This is valid to me. The following section is to help dispel the fear of *an imagined end*, and to introduce the <u>good news of life everlasting</u>. Here are some items that will be discussed:

how fears developed	etheric body
describe the next world	thought (mind) reading
no need for possessions	emotional links
spiritual development	reason for negatives
the Law of Karma	the rewards

In dealing with death, we need to understand that the body is the instrument we use to express life on earth. When the body ends its function, that does not mean that our life dies. You are *you* and will go on being you when the Spirit leaves the body. You need not fear this event any more than you fear going to sleep tonight.

The transition into another dimension is an eternal step we all take at the appropriate time. To be fearful of this or to deny it is to be unrealistic. One declares faith in the intelligence of the universe and eternal life, and achieves subsequent peace of mind. This maturity brings wisdom and a blessed soul.

Everything on earth vibrates with spirit. Spirit is the essence of life in every blade of grass, every leaf, every Oak or Sequoia that rises to blue sky. Vibration is in the enormous wind as well as the silent desk. It is in animals... plants, rivers and mountains, roads and bridges...your car, and even your toaster over. Spirit vibrates in *all*.

Don't underestimate the Spirit. You will not pass on until your purpose here is finished, and your own spirit is ready to go on. As you trust God's guidance in this world, know that the same Presence and Power will be with you eternally, preparing your way in love and wisdom.

<u>Some Basic Work to be Done</u>. There are many negatives in the human experience. People are hurt and disappointed, lose jobs, lose loved ones, see their dreams fade away. Yet----*a transformation needs to happen.* Over time, the challenges and pain are removed. But not necessarily the same for everyone.

This transformation is very personal; it is different for each soul. The individual seeks Truth to recover from the difficulties... to learn how to forgive, first himself/herself, then all others where there have been anger, resentment, jealousy, and other deleterious emotions.

As a person seeks the truth of their own life, there is a reward. That reward is health, harmony, prosperity, joy and happiness, a sense of their power, and a loving heart.

Time is a great variable. The achievement of change and growth may take a large segment of time or a small one. It depends on the individual. When one discovers a path that appears to improve their life, they can ignore it or become energetic and happily continue. They develop a spiritual understanding and open the way for guidance that helps their circumstances. The wise, intuitive, and sincere person can find wonderful, innovative solutions… aspects of living… if they concentrate hard enough.

How and Why Fear Developed. Certain invalid teaching occurred in past centuries, in which young people were taught to fear death in disciplining them into good conduct. They were taught to regard death with dread. Such fear seems to dissipate at age 35-40, but many people have such fear all of their lives.

Do not reject fear. A feeling of fear is simply protection of the body. All of our feelings are valid. A feeling of pain is God's way of indicating that a change is needed. A feeling of hate tells us that we have an attraction to something that we fear. A feeling of grief tells us that we are attached to an experience that we have outgrown. A feeling of despair makes us give up some rigid attitude that we have and need to let go of.

You see the pattern? The feelings that we experience say this: **Don't be so inflexible; be willing to change!** Everything changes all the time, so go with it. You will be happier. You will like yourself more. And your wife or husband or partner, children, mother-in-law, friends, boss, and neighbor will, too.

What Is It Like In The Next World?

There is absolutely no reason to fear death. There *is* no death. Fear of the unknown is real, yet unnecessary. When a person appears to die, all that happens is that he leaves his body here and goes on to the next place. He falls asleep here and wakes up on the other side; he is now Spirit, a cloud-like, billowy entity, like surrealism or impressionistic art. In many instances, it is easier than being born.

In this Earth world, we use the physical body for basic transportation. In New York we walk or take a cab or ride the subway; in L.A., we drive a car. We might move a lot... different apartments, houses, and jobs. Maybe different partners. We take everything so seriously here. It seems that there aren't enough smiles or laughter to go around. (Except with children.) Life has value, reason, and purpose. But mostly, it is a school. And we are trying to get good grades!

We continue to talk about the next world and refer to *God Given, Answers To Your Questions.* This discussion is about understanding eternity. The author states, "The body is outerwear, not your home. It is temporary housing to be treated with respect while in the life. In the moment of transition, you no longer need a body, so you discard it.... and you are lifted up. This is a doorway; a portal of sorts, to transport you as you float through it."

No living being actually dies, but continues on, into new dimensions and expressions. The spiral of life is upward.

It is clear to me that there are various opinions, deep feelings and beliefs of spiritually-endowed people----those who have had near death experiences, authors or intellectuals, and those who are scientists or researchers----all of whom have given a great deal of thought to the subject of the afterlife. I have studied and written this book with the desire to learn about eternal life, to build concepts about life, immortality, and the soul. To say that it is fascinating is a vast understatement.

In the next world, it may be a happy place. There is a joyful atmosphere as the transition takes place. You will be greeted by friends and family who are glad to see you. From what I've read, they are delighted when we return home.

At the moment of the transition, there is a step-up of energy; an increase in speed. You are vibrating faster than before. There is a shift in your consciousness. If there is pain, it is normal to want to live. But the body changes; the physical form is left behind. Feeling and movement go away. There is no pain at the moment of death.

Then, silence, and peace. You still exist. The biggest surprise is that dying does not end life.

Note---I am indebted to P.M.H. Atwater, Ph.D., author of 15 books, who wrote a profound book entitled, "*Dying to Know You.*" I used this book for reference, particularly for NDE (near death experiences). The author is a world authority; she has addressed audiences far and wide, including the United Nations.

Atwater writes, "At death, you can still think, you can still see, hear, move, reason, and wonder… It is different; you no longer have a dense body to filter and amplify the various sensations you had. Nothing is lost; you are not your body."

We have two bodies, the physical body we know so well, and a second body made of ether. You cannot see the etheric body. The two bodies are sort of attached; you will understand why in a moment. Each body has a different vibration rate. When you are awake, the two bodies are connected, but when you fall asleep, the etheric slips away from the physical body.

This slipping away happens if you are unconscious or under anesthesia… or are asleep. The etheric body has all your thoughts and feelings, including the conscious and the subconscious minds. The etheric body holds your human personality. The physical body begins to decay upon transition, while the etheric carries the personality over.

The etheric body passes into the next dimension after leaving the physical form. It is like waking up. The new life has begun. There is a sense of well-being and youth, which is surprising and pleasant to an elderly person. There are new colors and sounds, which are more exciting than what we have here. In the next world, thought *or mind* reading is the normal method of communication; thoughts are read immediately. There is no deception... and there are no old people on the other side. The full use of one's faculties are returned.

***

To conclude, I want to list some of the references I have used, with much appreciation to these authors: *Power Through Constructive Thinking* (Emmet Fox); *Dying to Know You* (P.M.H. Atwater, Ph.D.); *Emmanuel's Books II, III* (Pat Rodegast, Judith Stanton); *God Beyond Religion* (George Bockl); *The Gospel of Emerson* (Newton Dillaway); *God Given, Answers To Your Questions* (Denise Bennett, Ph.D.); *Timeless Secrets of Health and Rejuvenation* (Andreas Moritz); *Your Mind Can Heal You* (Frederick Bailes); *Proof of Heaven* (Eben Alexander); *The Seat of the Soul* (Gary Zukav); *Conversations With God* (Neal Donald Walsch); *Journey With the Master* (Eva Bell Werber).

No Need For Possessions. Here on earth we build up a certain character and mentality, based on our thinking and acting. In the next world, we will gravitate to where we belong and with those of similar interests. After a period of getting used to the new world, people have a great sense of well-being and an interesting life. It is different; money does not exist because there is no need for possessions. What you can think of clearly, you simply have.

The main difference between the two worlds is that things are instantaneous there; results come much more slowly here.

As to meeting friends and relatives, if there was an emotional connection on earth, it is likely you will meet. But, related persons here on earth probably will not be related to you in the next world.

On the next plane, there are many opportunities to broaden intellect and philosophical understanding. On earth we seem to have little understanding about life... why we are here, why there is such turmoil and fear, and why love is so fleeting. So many questions and so few answers.

On *this* plane, (Earth), we focus on money, success in our work or business, promotions, food and fun, social activities, possessions, etc. In the next world, none of these things have any meaning.

Over time, the physical desires that a person felt in life fade away. The individual, who has made an effort to live in a positive manner in thought and action, who has been kind and thoughtful to others----and contributed in some way----has the possibility of a rewarding experience in the next dimension.

Spiritual Development. Chapter 18 provides discussion on spiritual development, and I add a thought or two here: A life on Planet Earth is a matter of great choice, reflecting parental influence and training, the spiritual experiences drawn from religious teachings, and other opportunities as we seek a belief system to satisfy yearnings of the spirit. The effort of seeking is commendable, and it sometimes takes a lifetime of study to get answers.

Here is a brief overview of the *12 laws of karma. 1. The Law of Cause and Effect.* Karma is action or deed and refers to a principle where the actions of an individual bring a reaction for that person's future. *You reap what you sow. 2. The Law of Creation.* We create what we want; simple enough. *3. The*

Law of Humility. If we are humble and can accept others, then we can accept things as they are. *4. The Law of Growth*. We grow by accepting internally. *5. The Law of Responsibility*. The outside world responds to how we accept our obligations and responsibilities. *6. The Law of Connection*. This is how we connect the past to the present. *7. The Law of Focus*. This reflects how we focus on one thing at a time; it is a valued action. *8. The Law of Giving*. The habits of our giving reflect our beliefs and generosity. *9. The Law of Change.* This enables us to gain new and strong energies. *10. The Law of Here and Now*. We are wise to follow this law by living in the *present*. *11. The Law of Patience* brings its own reward. Lastly, *12. The Law of Inspiration*. Our contribution to life that benefits from our attention brings positive karmic results.

Here is an example of karmic law at work: A man, let us say, in Philadelphia, has a personality that is mean; he takes advantage of others. This is considered a karmic imbalance of energy. He will be taken advantage by others to <u>balance the energy</u>. If it can't be done in this life, it will occur in another. The karmic debt must be paid.

Reincarnation and karma work together to provide lessons for the soul to learn. If our actions cause sorrow in another person, we will feel that sorrow in this lifetime or the next. And if we bring harmony and love to another, we will feel that harmony and love.

There are individuals that are selfish and hostile, but we can't always know why they are that way. It is a mystery. If a person excessively punishes a child, that treatment is unfair; such behavior is part of their karmic connection. Zukav writes that healthy and balanced souls are incapable of harming others.

<u>The Reason For Negatives.</u> Every difficult thing that happens in life has purpose; every encounter is valid, whether

good or bad. Every rejection... every time something occurs in life that is considered negative... all is within the framework of lessons to be learned. Negatives show our lack of ability to realize Spirit; they are a signal for another step to be made in our growth and understanding.

Our Soul----the spiritual essence of a human being, the entity that sets the physical body in motion and provides life----is the piece of God in you. Not every person believes the same when it comes to the great mysteries of life. But it need not close the door just because we don't understand. The door I refer to is opportunity to learn, to gain **wisdom.**

Mostly, I feel that the negative incidents and events that come around are there to get our attention, to manifest a change in our behavior. Eventually----not necessarily a day later, or a year or a specific time, but *eventually*----you will see that the devastation that occurred was one of the best things that could ever happen to you. "There are no moments that ought not to have happened," wrote Pat Rodegast and Judith Stanton. "Nothing comes about by chance."

Here's your homework: Look back in your past. List two or three incidents that were so serious, you will never forget them. Rate the event in terms of their emotional impact immediately after the happening. Use a scale of 1-10, 1 being rather unimportant, 10 being horrendous. Then rate the event as you feel that it was a valid lesson for you. Use 1 as not very important; use 10 as an extremely valuable lesson.

As we study about the higher realms, we review the system of vibrations. There are two basic types: the mind where lower forms of thought reside; and the mind where the thoughts are light.

In the first realm, heavy and dense vibrations involve hang-ups, addictions, fears, guilt, anger, regrets, self-pity, arrogance, and resentment. The mind stays in this blockage as long as it takes to modify the development and change to faster and lighter vibrations.

In the second realm, the vibrations recognize positive thoughts: abilities, joys, courage, generosity, caring, empathy, patience, thoughtfulness, and loving kindness.

Souls have the choice to move to the realm that is best for their highest good.

The rewards. What we are in the deepest part of ourselves is revealed in our personality and actions in this life. How we treat others – the efforts made to exhibit kindness, understanding, love and forgiveness – are determiners for future experiences. No particular religious, political, or social preferences make much difference. Individual will power and strong beliefs are causal factors in the rewards of lives. Modifying behavior, correcting unsuitable habits, and becoming more spiritual in our belief are most rewarding. ~

Chapter 18

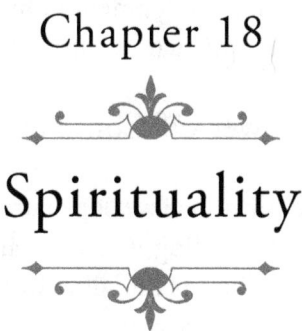

Spirituality

"WE ARE MADE in the image of God, not in the sense of physical appearance, but with respect to the power in our souls and the potential of our minds," wrote Atwater. In conclusion she wrote,

"We cannot keep the life on earth, not our possessions or relationships. What we can keep is our memories and our feelings of what we have integrated into our heart of hearts from the experience of being here, plus the love we have shared with others."

The word, "spirituality" is such a general, all-encompassing word. It means different things at different stages in our development. As we grow in wisdom, we are able to grasp more meaning in life. I've included some quotes here that hold special meaning for me.

Emmet Fox wrote, "The knowledge of Truth is its own reward, and that reward is health, harmony, and prosperity, to begin with; but this is only the beginning. The real object of the seeker should be the development of his own faculties and powers; in a word, his Spiritual Evolution."

The Power Of Consciousness

All we do, all we are, all we believe, is a matter of consciousness. This is the system of deciding where we are going----that is, what we choose to do in our life, how we will accomplish it, who we will be with----every conceivable experience that will occur as long as we breathe. Not only that, but the afterlife believer will be making decisions that will probably be a part of future lives.

Now, is all of this guaranteed? Of course not. There are conditions. It depends on how one cares for their life. It is similar to the attention one pays to a partner, pet, car, or job. For the partner: share good food, take out occasionally, go dancing, loving and intimacy, communicating, buying flowers, travel, etc. For the pet: good food, petting, communicating with him, health check ups, etc. For the car: fuel, care and attention, (keeping it clean), talking to it, maintenance and repairs, etc. For the job: dedication and attention, good communication, respect, etc.

If an individual has integrity and strives for goals and qualities in life such as appreciation, belief in a friendly universe, love and respect for other humans, (and animals, trees, and nature), then he has an *awareness of spirituality* in his soul. His energy and influence are elevated to the joys that life can offer.

Everybody knows that the greatest gift in this world is love. When one expresses love, that gift is returned to him.

What goes around comes around. It is as old as the hills… and the essence of happiness.

Star Gazing And The Deity

Every night, after the activities of the evening and as we are about to go to bed, I take the trash out to the side yard. I look up and see a favorite star, and gaze at its brightness. And I think, it takes at least four years for its light to reach the earth, at *186,000 miles per second.*

Our sun is a medium-sized star. There are billions of stars in our galaxy… and millions of galaxies in the universe. Scientists say, there is probably more than one universe. And---- there are probably planets inhabited by humanoids.

How did the galaxies get here? Is there a Creator? Is there a God above? A profoundly intelligent man, Albert Einstein, said that the universe functions by Intelligence, Nature, and Thought.

We human beings cannot fully comprehend the concept of the Deity. We are all bodies, minds, and souls. As we attempt to understand how and why we are here, the beliefs we embrace are our possessions in mind and heart. They carry us through the joyful events and the vicissitudes; the big decisions and the trivial.

Long ago, I adopted this belief: *God is as near as our next breath.* We take more than 20,000 breaths a day!

I view this existence as a gift. What we do here and how we get along, what thoughts and attitudes we have, how we act----all of that is up to the individual. But the Creator – Spirit, God, Source – provides the gift.

Recently, I was discussing *intuition* with a friend. Most of our perception comes from sensory signals: hearing, seeing, touching, smelling, and tasting. Intuition is a communication with higher intelligence. Somewhere, somehow... there is a message which directs us in a helpful manner. Tap into it. Follow your hunches. But----it is still your good judgment that must apply to determine if your hunch is right for you.

Impulse, insight, and feeling come into play as your subconscious mind or soul, may be signaling you. In the final analysis of every event, every act and deed in your life, it is your life! You may not believe it, but you have the control.

Human beings are complex creatures. We must take care of the body. It requires proper food, rest, nutrition, and the other essentials. We need to deal with the intellect; it can take us far in our daily progress. Then there's our soul. It has great power as to our past, present, and future, and a connection with the universe.

In this book, we have emphasized how thoughts create the conditions of our lives. Thoughts have a *cause and effect* power, and they create our emotions and the quality of our life. As we seek happiness, we can rely on our thoughts to become words, then actions, and reactions. Never think that you are stuck in an unhappy place; it is only temporary. Begin digging yourself out as soon as you can.

You already have the solution in your mind to every problem. You are the master of the circumstances of your life.

Spiritual Understanding: Health, Harmony, and Prosperity

What is spiritual understanding? It is an awakening; it is developing the Self, the evolving of one's faculties and powers, thereby bringing many qualities of a good life. One's *spirit* is the non-physical part of them. Spirit is the seat of the emotions, the heart and character... deep-down beliefs. It is the *Soul, which is said to be able to survive physical death or separation.* In life, we seek to achieve harmony between our physicality and our spirit. Mostly, this would be evidenced by our thoughts and our attitudes, and how we get along with others.

As one acquires this understanding, the circumstances of their life improves, and they enjoy better health and harmony. It is my belief that reaching out to people with the effort to be kind and thoughtful can sometimes result in pleasant things that come your way. Not always---but sometimes.

Random acts of kindness, where one pays for a toll for the car behind them, or a stranger's breakfast, or similar surprise---- brings some great smiles and fun.

A spiritual connection to a Creator, a Cosmic Intelligence, a divine system or universal order, sets us as spiritual beings, not robots. We are so much more.

We are spiritual beings having a human experience. And there's more... we are creatures of love. We can do kind things, be generous, share thoughts, be polite, and meet responsibilities. But the essence of our humanity – the basis of our nature – is love.

Our frustrations and challenges sometimes monopolize our time, leaving little left for the expression of love in our hearts. There are different kinds of love, represented by the gods of Ancient Greece... *Eros*: romantic, passionate love; *Philia*: intimate, authentic friendship; Ludus: playful, flirtatious love; *Storge*: unconditional, familial love; *Philautia*: self-love; *Pragma*: committed, companionate love; *Agape*: universal love.

These are Greek terms for various types of love. If one embraces the world and believes in the friendliness of the universe, it is *Agape* love. Love for the family would be *Storge* love. A deep friendship would be *Philia* love. A wonderful, passionate love for your partner would be *Eros* love.

And we can't forget the incredible love of pets, which provides us with a unique experience as we watch beautiful, loving creatures capture human hearts.

The Physical and the Spiritual

Almost everything we do in a typical day involves the physical... waking up, turning off the alarm, getting breakfast, going to work, and doing our duties. The spiritual is different; it is a sense of connecting to something bigger than ourselves. Spirituality involves a search for meaning in life. It is a universal human experience.

We think about our existence and ask, "Why are we in this life?" We may examine our thinking and beliefs about the mysteries of the universe. We are always trying to get answers that are beyond human understanding. It is an opportunity to look beyond the physical, to see perspectives that might help somehow to give us deeper awareness. And maybe some emphasis and insights on love.

We know that love is very important; we have been told that all our lives. There are only two religions: fear or love.

Our greatest enemy is fear. Fear is energy that contracts. Love is energy that expands.

It is in the stars. We are made of the same stuff as the stars. Scientists tell us about the formations that occurred millions of years ago. The history of human beings, 10,000 years ago, is revealed to us to give understanding. We set the information to words and stories to enhance the meaning.

The kings, the religionists, the philosophers, the writers, the poets, all seek the truth. But there is no acceptable evidence.

There is only faith. There are two reasons that every person has faith. First, because we are not falling off the earth, and second, because it is impossible to believe that the stars, planets, and galaxies simply appeared with no creative intelligence.

Yet, we want to know if creation has a Creator, thus introducing _love_ to the story... for life without love and truth is not beauty. Keats wrote, "That is all you know, and all you need to know."

Life is eternal; we need to learn this, and dwell in joy, not fear; in love, not hate; in acceptance, not hostility. As long as there is breath in us, we will search for meaning, and that means love and happiness. It all blends together for our good.

I suspect that the Creator wants it that way.~

Epilogue

EVERYONE WANTS HEALTH and happiness in their life. In this book, I attempted to define some ways to achieve these things. Some people look so joyful; they smile and seem so light-hearted in everything they do; others are doom-and-gloom types.

Achieving happiness is a science – an art. It is an awareness of psychology. In science there are specific acts or behaviors. Art would require creativity, and psychology would need emotional perception.

Each life is unique… complex, and emotionally impacted with its special qualities and style. Also, the factor of change is a constant. There is no life without challenge, negativity, and loss.

Why is that? Because we are here to grow socially, intellectually, physically, emotionally, and spiritually. And that cannot be accomplished by discussion; it is done by experience. It occurs by living more than a single life. You will come to understand that love heals everything, that there is a Universal Intelligence that provides guidance through the existence of the soul.

The personality of each individual has unique characteristics, which determine what we do, who we love, whether there are children, the circumstances of our lives, the intriguing possibilities of grace, bliss, joy beyond our wildest dreams, and health, wealth, and wisdom.

You opened this book, perhaps wondering if you could find happiness in your life. You may have discovered some new ideas. I say that you deserve happiness, good health, and wealth, too.

May your relationships be pleasant and joyful, through the changes that occur over time, and that you benefit in your social and emotional experiences.

Life is eternal, and we need to learn this, and dwell in faith, not fear; love, not hate; friendship, not hostility. We need to treasure this planet that we share and embrace our time here, in a caring atmosphere.

Let us honor the stars and galaxies, and respect our loved ones and ourselves as well. ~

CPSIA information can be obtained
at www.ICGtesting.com
Printed in the USA
BVHW090759201120
593719BV00015B/1032